READY REVIEW FOR THE GENERAL SURGERY ORAL BOARDS

BENJAMIN WEI, M.D.

This book is not intended for clinical use. The author and publishers are not responsible for errors or omissions in the book itself or from any consequence from application of the information of the book and make no warranty, expressed or implied, with respect to the currency, completeness, or accuracy of the contents of the publication. Application of this information remains the professional responsibility of the practitioner.

Information contained in this book was obtained from a review of current surgical textbooks, cancer treatment guidelines, and board study guides. The American Board of Surgery does not sponsor or endorse this book.

Back cover: Statue of Asklepios, Greek god of medicine and healing, Museo Pio-Clementino (Musei Vaticani). Image courtesy of the VROMA Project (www.vroma.org).

Foreword

Looking back at my residency, I felt that 90% of my clinical time was devoted to perhaps 25% of the material that the American Board of Surgery Certifying Exam covers. I believe that this booklet covers the highlights of the remaining information in a concise, high-yield format that through concentrated studying will allow you to demonstrate this knowledge reflexively in the high-pressure, time-limited setting that is the oral board exam. The management of conditions often encountered by the typical general surgeon is not covered, in the interest of space and time. The material has been distilled from a multitude of sources, including most uniquely, I believe, the latest NCCN guidelines. It will not be an easy read, at a dense 60 pages or so, but if you know the information cold, I believe you will be much more comfortable dealing with board scenarios that are uncommonly encountered in clinical practice.

In addition, I have included key pointers for nearly all the procedures listed in Zollinger's classic, the Atlas of Surgical Operations. I was asked how to perform the majority of the operations that were discussed during the course of my exam. Again, I have not included much detail on the more common operations that each of us has probably done numerous times.

Please do send me your comments and suggestions for how to improve this guide. I hope you find yourself as prepared as you can be when you face your examiners on game day.

Benjamin Wei
benjaminweimd@gmail.com
October 2011

How to use this book

In addition to using this book, I suggest purchasing the latest edition of John Cameron's **Current Surgical Therapy**, which is invaluable as a reference text. Marc Neff's book, **Passing the General Surgery Oral Board Exam**, is also helpful for reviewing the most common board scenarios. Going through mock orals, either at your institution or at a course such as Osler, should increase your familiarity with the format of the exam and improve your confidence. This text focuses on clinical topics that are probably tested more than they are seen in "real life"; a review of entities such as small bowel obstruction and cholecystitis should probably be sought elsewhere.

My advice is to read and reread this book at least a few times, preferably both weeks ahead of time and shortly before the exam. The operative guide, I believe, especially deserves a reread right before the exam. There are a quite a few abbreviations, a guide to which is located at the end of the book.

For the sake of brevity, T staging for cancers of the alimentary tract is not described under each subtopic – as a general rule, and unless otherwise noted, T1 cancers are limited to the mucosa/submucosa, T2 cancers extend into but not through the muscle, T3 cancers penetrate through the muscle but not past the adventitia, and T4 cancers invade adjacent organs. As further clarification, the notation "T1+" means any cancer staged T1 or greater (the same shorthand applies to nodal staging).

TABLE OF CONTENTS

HEAD/NECK

Parotid tumors – CT or MRI neck, FNA to r/o benign non-epithelial pathology (ex. LN, lipoma, lymphoepithelial lesion → no sx), then proceed with superficial parotidectomy w/ frozen. If benign → nothing additional. If low-grade malignant → XRT. If high-grade malignant → radical parotidectomy +/- resection of facial nerve, MRND, XRT.

Cancer in cervical LN, unknown primary – 1st get CXR (eval for lung ca, mediastinal LAN, TB, sarcoid). If +URI then observe w/ abx x 2 wks. Then FNA: 1) if SCC →excisional bx, CT neck/chest, EGD, laryngoscopy, bronch, EUA mouth/larynx → if no primary: MRND/XRT; 2) if adenocarcinoma → excisional bx, CT neck/chest/abdomen pelvis, EGD, colonoscopy, mammograms → if no primary: MRND with possible XRT; 3) if thyroid ca → total thyroidectomy with LND of enlarged nodes if papillary/follicular, CLND/MRND if medullary; 4) if melanoma → MRND, excise primary, superficial parotidectomy if lesion on upper face (ie. cancer has crossed parotid on way to cervical LN)

Branchial cleft cyst – 1st: located at base of ear or angle of mandible, passes facial nerve; 2nd (most common): anterior border SCM, passes between carotid bifurcation into palatine tonsil; 3rd: lower border of SCM, passes behind carotid through thyrohyoid membrane to enter larynx; 4th (extremely rare): lateral neck, follows course of recurrent laryngeal nerve to enter piriform sinus

Head/neck SCC – staging: I=<2 cm, II=2-4 cm, III=>4 cm or +LN, IV=distant met; rx: stage I-II → WLE with 1-1.5 cm margin and XRT if microinvasion or suspicious for LN invasion by location (ex. intraoral) vs XRT 6000 rads if not resectable 2/2 location; stage III → WLE + MRND, postop XRT

THYROID/PARATHYROID

Standard thyroid workup – PE, USG, thyroid scan, thyroid function tests (TSH, T4, T3), anti-thyroperoxidase ab, anti-thyroglobulin ab, anti-Tg receptor ab screen, FNA

Non-toxic goiter – dx: CT if compression, PFTs/barium swallow prn for respiratory symptoms/dysphagia; rx: evaluate any suspicious/growing nodules w/ FNA; if symptomatic goiter, consider radioactive iodine or surgery

Chronic lymphocytic thyroiditis (Hashimoto's) – dx: +antithyroid antibodies (esp antithyroperoxidase); rx: evaluate any dominant nodule w/ FNA, thyroid replacement prn

Subacute granulomatous (de Quervain's) thyroiditis – dx: painful, hyperthyroid → hypothyroid → euthyroid, elevated ESR, elevated thyroglobulin, decreased RAIU, no bx needed; rx: NO antithyroid drugs, use beta-blockers, pain control, prednisone if severe (if does not respond to steroids question the diagnosis)

Subacute lymphocytic thyroiditis – dx: can be postpartum or sporadic; NOT painful, elevated thyroglobulin, decreased RAIU, no bx needed; rx: NO antithyroid drugs, use beta blockers

Acute suppurative thyroiditis – dx: neck pain/fluctuant mass, normal thyroid function tests, RAIU normal or cold, CT neck, FNA best test; rx: surgical drainage, possible lobectomy, appropriate abx (r/o fungal, TB w/ cx, parasites such echinococcus, strongyloides w/ serology, if +AIDS → eval for CMV, PCP, MAI)

Riedel's (fibrous) thyroiditis – dx: FNA/lobectomy to differentiate from thyroid cancer; rx: steroids, surgical resection if compressive

Grave's disease – dx: hyperthyroid (exophthalmos and pretibial myxedema are specific), diffusely elevated RAIU, +ab to TSH receptor; rx options: PTU/methimazole (no methimazole if pregnant), radioactive iodine but avoid for Grave's opthalmopathy(worsens)/kids/pregnant women, surgery; preop prep: make euthyroid with antithyroid meds, beta blockade if symptomatic, potassium iodide or Lugol's 10-14 days prior to surgery

Thyroid storm – rx: o2, IVF, steroids, beta-blockade, PTU, cooling blankets, sedatives

Toxic multinodular goiter – rx options: RAI (meds less effective), surgery; preop prep: same as Grave's, except NO iodine (exacerbates hyperthyroidism)

Solitary toxic nodule – dx: rarely (<1%) cancer; rx: thyroid suppression, RAI, antithyroid meds, surgery (if other treatments are ineffective/undesirable or if local effects/growth is seen)

Amiodarone-associated thyrotoxicosis – stop amio, RAI/antithyroid meds usually NOT effective, rx = surgery

Papillary thyroid ca – total thyroidectomy if PTC > 1 cm, or < 1 cm but multicentric or other mets (though in clinical practice usually perform total to permit RAI and f/u w/ thyroglobulin levels), if + clinical LNs perform CLND and MRND prn

Follicular thyroid neoplasms – thyroid lobectomy if adenoma, total thyroidectomy if invasive (ie. carcinoma), contralateral nodule > 1 cm, or hx of head/neck radiation; NO frozen section (cannot diff b/t adenoma or carcinoma – difference is presence of capsular invasion in carcinoma), if + clinical LNs (uncommon - < 5%) perform CLND/MRND prn

Staging for differentiated (ie. papillary/follicular) thyroid ca – if age < 45, stage I=M0, stage II=M1; if age > 45, stage I=T1(<2 cm), II=T2(2-4 cm), III=T3(>4 cm) or N1a (central LNs), IV=T4(invasive into adjacent structures),N1b(cervical/med LNs), or M1

Hurthle cell cancer – more often multifocal/bilateral/regional mets (compared to papillary or follicular), rx=total thyroidectomy with CLND, do MRND if clinical +LNs

Postop management papillary/follicular thyroid ca s/p total thyroidectomy – thyroid replacement, then make hypothyroid by withdrawing rx and give RAI 30 mCi, repeat dose in 6-12 months if residual uptake (NO need for RAI rx if unifocal papillary ca < 1 cm with no spread/mets), suppress TSH with thyroid hormone, XRT if incomplete surgical excision or extrathyroidal/LN spread, NO chemo, follow TSH/thyroglobulin levels, if elevated Tg level perform neck USG, whole-body thyroid scan and give RAI 150-200 mCi, consider resection/XRT if Tg levels fail to respond to RAI (depending on site)

Medullary thyroid ca – dx: amyloid on FNA, r/o MEN syndromes (send ca and urine catechols etc to r/o hyperparathyroidism and pheochromocytoma), also familial MTC (both + for RET mutation), check calcitonin (to dx recurrence)/CEA levels (for prognosis), if clinically +LNs or calcitonin > 400 check CTNCAP, rx=total thyroidectomy with CLND, and MRND prn for grossly or CT positive LNs; adjuvant=NO RAI (b/c no radiouptake), NO suppression dosing of thyroid hormone, XRT if positive margins/high-volume disease; f/u=calcitonin/CEA/neck USG, DMSA scan, CTC/MRI liver/bone scan if elevated calcitonin; recurrent or met disease rx = resect if feasible, otherwise options include dacarbazine-based chemo, XRT, experimental rx (ex. vandetanib – EGFR/VEGFR antagonist)

MEN2A (= medullary thyroid ca/ pheo/parathyroid hyperplasia)/**FMTC**→prophylactic thyroidectomy by 3-5 yrs (no CLND unless +nodule/LN mets); **MEN2B** = medullary thyroid ca/pheo/mucosal neuroma/Marfanoid → prophylactic thyroidectomy 1st year

Anaplastic thyroid ca – dx: CT neck/chest; rx: XRT/chemo (paclitaxel) +/- trach

Thyroid lymphoma – dx: may mimic anaplastic ca, suspect in Hashimoto's w/ enlarging goiter, proceed from FNA or core → open bx (to send for flow cytometry); rx=CHOP, if MALT lymphoma XRT alone

Indications for parathyroidectomy in asymptomatic PHPT – calcium > 1 above upper limit of normal, CrCl < 60, bone densitometry T score < 2.5 or previous fx, age < 50 yrs. Localize before exploration with: USG or CT neck/chest or sestamibi.

Missing parathyroid gland - If missing superior gland → search behind larynx, behind esophagus, carotid sheath, thyroid USG/lobectomy. If missing inferior gland → search above positions but also resect cervical thymus. If missing gland still, bx gland. If bx reveals parathyroid hyperplasia, remove 3 glands and CRYOPRESERVE in case pt truly only has 3 glands, then can reimplant if becomes hypocalcemic. If bx shows NO parathyroid hyperplasia, close, f/u PTH/Ca levels, obtain imaging for persistent HPT (see below) and explore accordingly. If repeat imaging all negative, consider referring to Endocrine specialist for possible repeat neck exploration.

Persistent/recurrent HPT – repeat imaging (sestamibi, USG, CT neck/chest), get selective venous sampling if other studies unrevealing (check PTH levels in SVC/IJVs looking for 2x step up), rule out familial hypocalciuric hypercalcemia w/ 24 hr urine calcium

Secondary HPT = parathyroid hyperplasia 2/2 hypocalcemia due to CRI; medical rx: limit phos intake, phos binders, HD → if persistent high PTH use calcitriol; rx: indications for sx – calciphylaxis, PTH > 600 in ESRD, Ca xPO > 55, cystic/fibrotic bone marrow, extraskeletal calcification; sx = total parathyroidectomy and reimplantation; postop – hungry bone syndrome (increased skeletal ca deposition, severe hypocalcemia)

Tertiary HPT = persistent parathyroid hyperplasia/hypercalcemia s/p renal transplant (95% resolve secondary HPT s/p renal transplant but may take 2 years to do so). Rx: sx indicated for severe hypercalcemia or symptoms/rising Cr; sx = total parathyroidectomy and reimplantation

BREAST

Cyclical mastalgia - r/o breast mass, breast infection, chest wall (ie. musculoskeletal) syndrome, pregnancy, get mammo if indicated; rx=primrose oil, anti-inflammatories, cessation of caffeine/chocolate, heat, tamoxifen, low-fat diet

Fibroadenoma – surgery if >2-3 cm, growing, painful

Breast cyst – USG first. If partly solid, rx as suspicious mass (ie. core bx followed by excision prn). If completely liquid, aspirate. If clear and completely drained → observe, may aspirate again if recurs but excise if recurs twice. If clear but not completely drained, or bloody → excisional bx.

Phyllodes tumor – excise w/ 1 cm margin, NO ALND, if metastatic tends to go to lungs

Positive ALN with occult primary – dx: FNA → adenocarcinoma, excise (send for ER/PR → if + suggests breast ca, send for mucin → if + suggests GI ca), mammo, breast MRI if mammo negative, CXR (r/o lung primary), CTAP (r/o abdominal primary), bone scan (r/o bone met), EGD/colonoscopy (r/o GI primary); rx: if axillary histology + for breast AND no breast primary, ALND (preceded by neoadjuvant chemo if fixed/bulky) + then whole breast XRT withOUT mastectomy; if primary located, treat accordingly

DCIS – classifications: comedo vs non-comedo, low/intermediate/high grade depending on nuclear morphology and mitotic index; rx = BCT w/ XRT (+ SLNBx if large, palpable, high-grade, microinvasive) or mastectomy w/ SLNBx (do SLNBx b/c if you don't and +cancer in mastectomy specimen you've committed her to complete ALND). Prefer mastectomy if DCIS is multicentric, large, central, inadequate margins after BCT (can attempt re-resection x1), pt preference, + fam hx, contraindication to radiation; adjuvant rx=tamoxifen; recurrence rx=if prior BCT → mastectomy; if prior mastectomy → resect with negative margin and XRT if not contraindicated or previously given.

LCIS – if core needle bx positive → surgical excisional bx, but no need for re-resection if positive surgical margin; rx: observation (CBE, mammo annually) and tamoxifen (premenopausal) or raloxifene (postmenopausal), offer prophylactic bilateral mastectomy if +BRCA/strong family hx.

Paget's disease - 95% have underlying breast cancer; if unilateral nipple lesion, suspect Paget's and get CBE/USG/mammo (NO steroids), if no mass → excise NAC and if +Paget's cells → TM → if cancer, ALND; if mass present → excise NAC/excisional bx of mass → MRM if cancer, TM/SLNBx if DCIS. If bilateral skin changes of nipple more likely to be eczema.

Nipple discharge - if clear or galactorrhea → hCG, TSH (can be caused by hypothyroidism), prolactin level (if elevated get head MRI → if +prolactinoma rx w/ cabergoline/bromocriptine 1st, transsphenoidal hypophysectomy for failure of med mgmt); if bloody/colored → d/c caffeine/smoking, get imaging (mammo/USG), try to establish responsible quadrant w/ 6 wk period of observation. If can find responsible quadrant, perform wedge subareolar ductal excision; if no responsible quadrant, perform complete subareolar ductal excision. Most likely dx = intraductal papilloma. If associated mass on exam/imaging, do excisional bx also.

Breast cancer screening – standard: age 40, annual CBE/mammo; high risk = +family or personal hx of breast ca, +BRCA mutation, prior XRT w/ breast in field, prior dx of ADH or LCIS → CBE q6mo, annual mammo/MRI, if +family hx start screening 5-10 yrs before dx in relative or age 25 if BRCA+

BRCA-1/BRCA-2 – indications for testing = pt or pt family member develops breast ca at age < 50, presence of synchronous cancers

BRCA-1 - poorly diff; ER/PR negative so insensitive to tamoxifen

BRCA-2 – increased breast ca risk in men, more likely to be well diff and ER/PR positive than BRCA-1 ca.

BRCA prophylactic rx - both have increased risk of breast ca (90% chance) and ovarian ca (20-40% chance). Offer prophylactic bilateral TM and if done w/ having kids or menopausal, oophorectomy. If decline TM, continue annual high-risk breast screen (see above). If decline or not eligible yet for oophorectomy, get annual transvag USG and CA125 level

BIRADS – 0 – incomplete, 1 – negative, 2 – benign, 3 – probably benign (6 mo interval screen), 4 – suspicious (BIOPSY), 5 – likely malignant, 6 – known malignancy

MRI in breast cancer – indications: presence of invasive lobular cancer, unknown primary cancer, BRCA+, multiple or multicentric breast cancer, screening s/p breast augmentation.

Breast cancer staging - evaluate primary w/ CBE/mammo/USG/MRI prn. Get CXR/LFTs/bone scan only if symptomatic or alkaline phosphatase elevated/CTAP only if LFTs elevated/brain MRI only if symptomatic. T1<2 cm, T2 2-5 cm, T3 > 5 cm, T4 – invading skin/chest wall; N1=1-3 +LNs, not matted/fixed, N2=4-9 +LNs or LNs matted/fixed, N3=>10 +LNs, supraclavicular/internal mammary/infraclavicular LN

Breast cancer surgery - BCT (2-3 mm margins, orient specimen) w/ SLNBx followed by XRT, or TM w/SLNBx. Completion ALND if SLNBx positive. Multicentric, large tumor, small breast, previous XRT, contraindication to XRT → favor mastectomy

SLNBx – indicated for T1-3, clinical N0 breast cancer, palpable/high-grade/extensive DCIS, and DCIS pts undergoing mastectomy; NOT for T4 or inflammatory breast ca (do ALND instead); results - macromet (>2 mm), micromet (0.2-2 mm) → completion ALND, isolated tumor cells (<0.2 mm) → no ALND

Neoadjuvant rx – indications: large (T3) tumor if considering BCT, locally invasive (T4 or N2+) disease or inflammatory breast cancer; rx = first, AC or TC or TAC, plus trastuzumab if Her2+ (give AFTER doxorubicin done); then, 1) if resectable → MRM → postop chemo + XRT; 2) if not resectable, add taxotere (if not given already) + XRT and reassess. Exception is that you CANNOT give chemo if breast ca has ulcerated through skin; give XRT and perform salvage MRM.

Adjuvant rx concepts – all pts should get endocrine therapy (tamoxifen if premenopausal and aromatase inhibitors if postmenopausal) – EVEN if ER/PR neg they have a small benefit; all Her2+ pts should get trastuzumab; >1 cm tumors and/or positive LNs are an indication for adjuvant chemo. Chemo is controversial in 0.5-1 cm tumor or tumor w/ micromets on LN bx. Do not give chemo in <0.5 cm tumors w/ NO micromets/mets to LNs.

Adjuvant XRT – which invasive BC pts get? All pts treated w/ BCT get XRT, also pts treated w/ MRM with positive nodes, large (> 5 cm=T3) tumors, close/positive margins should get XRT. In general MRM pts with negative LNs, small (<5 cm) size, good (>2-3 mm) margins do NOT get XRT. Remember you can only irradiate breast once; however if you have done XRT on one breast you CAN do XRT on the other side later.

Axillary XRT– give if ALND shows multiple (4+) positive axillary nodes.

Full metastatic workup (do for inflammatory breast cancer/recurrence/met) – CXR, CTCAP, bone scan, followed by PET if any of the above studies are positive/equivocal, if pt has metastatic disease perform brain MRI (PET not sensitive for brain mets)

Metastatic breast ca – consider resection of primary, XRT for bone/brain mets, consider metastectomy of lung/liver if isolated, assess receptors: if HER 2+/ER+ → trastuzumab + endocrine rx, if HER2+/ER- → trastuzumab + taxol, if HER2-/ER+ → endocrine rx, chemo for progression, if HER2-/ER- → chemo. Chemo = FAC + taxol.

Breast cancer in pregnancy - general concepts – no chemo in 1st trimester, no XRT during pregnancy, no tamoxifen during pregnancy, SLNBx OK with radionuclide but NOT blue dye;1st trimester → MRM + 2nd trimester chemo; late 1st trimester/2nd trimester → MRM or BCT (lumpectomy with SLNBx) + 2nd trimester chemo, post-birth XRT if indicated; 3rd trimester → MRM or BCT followed by chemo, post-birth XRT if indicated

Male breast cancer – dx: mammo/bx, also r/o liver disease (LFTs), sex-steroid producing tumor (hCG), Klinefelter's (low testosterone, gynecomastia, underdeveloped sexual characteristics, XXY), testicular abnormalities (PE); rx=MRM, also can do total mastectomy with SLNBx, BCT pointless, adjuvant XRT if large tumor/positive margins/4+ LNs, tamoxifen if ER+.

Aromatase inhibitors – one drug is anastrozole=arimidex –NOT for use in premenopausal women (actually will increase estrogen levels in these pts)

HER2+ → rx w/ trastuzumab = herceptin, +cardiotoxicity (hence don't use simultaneously w/ doxorubicin which is also cardiotoxic).

LUNG/MEDIASTINUM

Solitary pulmonary nodule (< 3 cm)/lung mass (> 3cm) hx - ? smoking, previous ca; PE – lymphadenopathy, Horner's syndrome; dx: prior CXR (if no change in 2 years, likely benign), whole body PET-CT (rounded → more likely hamartoma or met, spiculated → more likely cancer), PFTs, perc/transbronchial bx if close to pleural surface or bronchus respectively (if benign dx on bx → observe, if non-diagnostic → surgical wedge bx, if malignant → see below)

Lung cancer - rx: no surgery in general if T4 (invasive of critical structures-ex. heart, great vessels, carina, esophagus, RLN), malignant effusion, pleural mets, or met elsewhere. If primary lung cancer on preop bx and acceptable PFTs (ppoFEV1 > 40% or 0.8L, DLCO > 40%)→ bronch, mediastinoscopy, if med negative then proceed w/ VATS or open lobectomy. If no preop diagnosis need wedge first, then proceed w/ lobectomy if +cancer on frozen. If med shows N2 disease (positive ipsilateral nodes) → abort lobe and give neoadjuvant chemo +/- XRT, then consider restaging/sx. If med shows N3 disease (positive contralateral nodes) → abort and give definitive chemo/XRT (NO sx). Superior sulcus (pancoast) tumor → gets neoadjuvant XRT/chemo followed by resection. Tumor invading chest wall → open lobectomy w/ chest wall resection (take rib above and below tumor, 3 cm lateral margins, usually gore-tex or other prosthetic reconstruction), neoadjuvant NOT necessity. Chemo=cisplatin-based.

Pulmonary metastasis – whole-body PET-CT in general 1st to r/o other mets, consider resection if path favorable (YES for sarcoma, colorectal, breast, melanoma; NO for pancreatic, gastric, esophageal), PFTs OK, primary controlled, no other mets (or other mets resectable), lung mets completely resectable; do not need bronch/med if suspicion is for met; rx=wedge resection(s) – single or multiple – possible lobectomy if deep.

Hemoptysis – resuscitate (IVF, T+C) and control airway: intubate prn and place bronchial blocker, position pt w/ bleeding side down, rigid bronch to clear blood and establish airway if not already intubated, CXR and CT chest if stable, then bronchial arteriogram (pulm arteriogram if bronchial a-gram negative), lobectomy = option of last resort.

Pneumothorax – consider VATS w/ bleb resection (resect apex of lung) and mechanical pleurodesis if 2nd episode, prolonged air leak (> 7 days), complete lung collapse, worrisome profession (ex. pilot, scuba diver), poor access to medical care

Seminoma – dx: need biopsy, normal AFP/HCG, elevated LDH; rx: XRT

Non-seminoma GCTs – dx: need biopsy, elevated AFP/HCG; rx: cisplatin-based chemo, sx for residual disease

Thymoma – I (capsule intact) → sx; II (capsular invasion) → sx +/- adjuvant XRT; resectable III (organ invasion)/resectable IVA (pleural/pericardial dissemination) → induction chemo, then sx, then XRT; IVB (lymphogenous/hematogenous met) and unresectable III or IVA → chemo and/or XRT; thymoma can cause myasthenia gravis, pure red cell aplasia, hypogammoglobulinemia

ESOPHAGUS

Barrett's - BE only – EGD q1-3 yrs, GERD rx; BE with LGD – EGD q6mos, GERD rx, referral for possible RFA; BE with HGD – RFA if not surgical candidate with EGD q3mo, otherwise discuss esophagectomy.

Esophageal anatomy - prox esophagus=16-24 cm, mid esophagus=24-32, distal esophagus=32-40; upper 2/3rds =R chest, lower 1/3rd = L chest; lower esophageal sphincter – inadequate pressure < 6 mm Hg, inadequate intraabdominal length < 2 cm.

Esophageal testing = barium swallow, EGD (omit if suspect Zenker's), manometry, pH probe (if need to analyze for GERD)

Motility disorders – achalasia ("birds beak," failure of LES to relax): medical rx (ca channel blockers, NTG, botox, +/- dilation) → if above fail, surgery (Heller myotomy w/ partial fundoplication or if end stage/megaesophagus, esophagectomy); diffuse/esophageal spasm (simultaneous contractions throughout) or nutcracker esophagus (high-amplitude contractions) → medical rx, avoid surgery (long esophageal myotomy=last, last resort); zenkers → transoral stapling (if you know about this) or diverticulectomy w/ cricopharyngeal myotomy

Esophageal perforation – dx: swallow (gastrografin followed by thin barium if gastro negative), CXR may show pleural effusion, PTX, pneumomediastinum; rx: NPO, IVF, foley, chest tube if +effusion, broad abx including antifungals, immediate OR (though may consider observation w/ NPO/abx if small, contained leak w/ no signs of sepsis/minimal symptoms) → thoracotomy on side of effusion/leak, repair perf in 2 layers over NGT even if >24 hrs, intercostal flap, wide drainage. Postop give TPN, abx, get swallow at 7 days. If very ill → can consider either T-tube w/ wide drainage/G/J tubes or diverting esophagostomy w/ wide drainage/G/J tubes. If mega-esophagus, stricture, or known ca → prefer esophagectomy,

Esophageal cancer: dx: whole-body PET-CT, EUS, EGD w/ bx, stress prn, PFTs prn, bronch if upper 1/3rd, TPN prn; staging: N1=1-2LNs, N2=3-6LNs,N3=7+LNs; neoadjuvant rx=5-FU/cisplatin/4500 rads for T2+ or N1+ (only non-candidates are T1N0); nonresectable=ca < 5 cm from cricopharyngeus, T4b (invasive into unresectable organs), bulky mediastinal lymphadenopathy (though judgment call – depends on age, response to therapy), distant lymphadenopathy/metastatic disease; adjuvant rx=observation only (no adjuvant) in pts w/ SCC and R0 resection (regardless of stage), pts w/ adenoca and T1-T2N0 lesions w/ R0 resection and no preop therapy; give chemo-XRT in any R1-R2 resections, node positive distal/GE-J cancers; consider adjuvant chemo +/- XRT in all others.

Caustic injury – dx: remember airway (laryngoscopy, bronch, intubate prn), barium swallow or CTCAP w/ oral contrast, early EGD (<24 hrs); grades: 1st degree=edema/hyperemia, 2nd degree=ulceration, 3rd degree=eschar with or without full-thickness necrosis; rx: all pts – NPO until pain free, IVF, PPI; 1st degree → observation; 2nd/3rd degree → ICU, abx, serial CXR, TPN, repeat esophagram at 48h and prn thereafter, go to OR if +perf/necrosis (esophagectomy w/ diverting esophagostomy, J tube), pts need f/u EGD/barium swallow b/c of risk of stricture (dilate prn, resection/reconstruction if recalcitrant)

Paraesophageal hernia – types: I=sliding, hiatal, II=GEJ correctly located, paraesophageal, III=GEJ above diaphragm, paraesophageal, IV=GEJ and other organs above diaphragm, paraesophageal; rx: I=repair if operating for GERD indication, II/III/IV=may cause anemia, repair even if asymptomatic.

STOMACH

H. pylori – azithromycin or amoxicillin + flagyl + PPI for 10-14 d, urea breath test best for verifying eradication. Rx x12 wks → EGD → 12 wks and repeat EGD, if refractory then may consider surgical therapy

Gastric lymphoma – stages: I-no LNs, II-perigastric/subdiaphragmatic LNs, III-supradiaphragmatic LNs, IV-distant disease; stages I-II: sx or chemo/XRT, stages III-IV: chemo-XRT only. Chemo=1) rituxan 2) CHOP.

Gastric ulcer – ALL need to be biopsied either intraop or post-procedure/op. Type II/III ulcers are acid hypersecretors and may benefit from vagotomy w/ antrectomy or pyloroplasty (esp if hx of PUD rx already). Factors predicting failure endoscopic therapy – visible vessel, ulcer > 2 cm deep, deep posterior, >4 units prbcs; rx: bleeding → angio, if refractory, then wedge or suture ligation/bx; perforated→ wedge or Graham patch/bx. Can consider V+ A if low-risk pt, stable, hx of PUD refractory to meds.

Refractory ulcer after anti-ulcer sx – dx: old records, EGD, h. pylori, UGIS, gastrin, secretin-stimulated gastrin level, calcium, technetium scan (if +, retained antrum), sham feeding test (measure BAO, SAO w/ chewing steak, PAO w/ pentagastrin stim – BAO > 2 mmol/h or SAO/PAO > 10% = inadequate vagotomy), steak meal test (gastrin incr >200-300% → antral G cell hyperplasia, may see smaller increase w/ retained antrum)

PUD sx complications – dumping syndrome → somatostatin, small meals, convert to RYGJ prn; post-vagotomy diarrhea → lomotil, somatostatin, cholestyramine, decr fluid intake, reversed jejunal interposition prn; alkaline gastritis → cholestyramine, reglan, convert to RYGJ prn; post-surgical gastroparesis → reglan, erythromycin, antrectomy (if no previous resection) or subtotal gastrectomy (if previous antrectomy) prn

Mallory-Weiss – PPI, vasopressin, EGD w/ therapy, angio, operate if all of the above fail, NO blakemore/minnesota tube

Stress gastritis – carafate, PPI, misoprostil, octreotide, vasopressin, EGD w/ therapy, angio, sx if failure: high risk → 4 vessel ligation w/ oversewing bleeders (leave short gastrics); low risk → subtotal gastrectomy w/ RYGJ

Zollinger-Ellison syndrome - dx: gastrin level (hold PPIs before checking, see hypergastrinemia w/ Z-E but also w/ achlorhydria – ex. pernicious anemia, atrophic gastritis – or w/ elevated acid secretion – ex. +h. pylori, GOO, G-cell hyperplasia, retained antrum, CRI), many false positive/negatives based on absolute level alone so also do secretin stim test (gastrin will go up s/p secretin in Z-E patient); 25% pts have MEN-I (**P**arathyroid, **P**ituitary, **P**ancreatic tumor); localization modalities: CTAP, MRI, octreotide scan, EUS; rx: resect (enucleate it in pancreas if does not involve duct, Whipple vs distal panc if it does), if cannot localize – kocherize, IOUS, open duodenum and palpate, if still cannot find do V +P, and give ZAP-5 – streptozosin, doxorubicin, PPI, 5-FU, somatostatin.

Gastric cancer – dx=EGD w/ bx, EUS; staging=CTCAP; rx: resect if no mets, distal or total gastrectomy w/ 6 cm margins, if near GEJ → Ivor-Lewis; neoadjuvant chemo w/ ECF (epirubicin, cisplatin, 5-FU) in pts with T2+N1+ cancer, neoadjuvant chemoXRT w/ 5-FU/cisplatin if GEJ tumors; adjuvant chemoXRT (5-FU based) in pts with any R1/R2 resection or R0 resection w/ T3+ or N1+ path, sometimes used in T2N0

GIST – dx: bx is c-kit+, sporadic, rare LN mets in adults, hypervascular, predictors of recurrence=mitotic rate, tumor size, tumor location; sx: 1-2 cm margins, no LAN; neoadjuvant=give if large, invasive/extensive, duodenal, low rectal, near GEJ; adjuvant rx: gleevec if >5 cm or high grade (>10 mitosis/hpf) – note: low grade is < 5 m/hpf, intermediate grade is 5-10 m/hpf; f/u=q3-6 mos CTAP for first 5 year, then annually; recurrence: repeat resection if possible, otherwise gleevec; if no response to gleevec → sunitinib (sutent)

Duodenal ulcer (bleeding) – rx: sx if >6 units prbcs, HD unstable, refractory to endoscopic rx.; high risk → suture ligation; low risk, small ulcer, no previous comps → suture ligation; low risk, large (>2 cm) or previous comps → V+A.

Duodenal ulcer (perforated) – rx: high risk, small (<2 cm) → Graham patch, high risk, large (> 2cm) → jejunal patch (NOT serosal, really = duodenojejunostomy); low risk, small → Graham patch or V + A including ulcer if hx of PUD/refractory to PPI; low risk, large → V + A.

Duodenal ulcer (obstructing): if no response to 7d of medical therapy (NGT, PPI, IVF, repeat UGIS) → gastrojejunostomy w/ parietal cell vagotomy (difficult to perform pyloroplasty or antrectomy in scarred/edematous duodenum)

SMALL BOWEL

Carcinoid – dx: chromogranin, 24 hr 5HIAA urine levels, EGD, colonoscopy, capsule study, CTAP, octreotide scan, TTE to r/o valvular disease, preop rx w/ octreotide prn carcinoid syndrome; sx: duodenal - <2 cm → transduodenal excision, >2 cm, into muscle, or LAN → whipple; rectal - <2 cm → local excision, > 2 cm/into muscle/LAN → APR; resect liver mets if possible (if not can try RFA, TACE, chemo-embolization); carcinoid syndrome: octreotide, 2nd line=IFN, if crisis → hydrocortisone, antihistamines, albuterol; chemo=streptozocin combinations.

ECF – dx: CTAP, fistulagram, output: low <200, moderate 200-500, high >500; rx: initially make NPO, attempt to feed enterally if does not significantly increase output, TPN otherwise, wound care/protect skin, perc drains prn, abx prn, observe x6 wks, plan for OR in 12-16 wks if failure to resolve. FRIENDS=foreign body, radiation, infection/IBD, epithelialization, neoplasia, distal obstruction.

Crohn's – medical rx: sulfasalazine/mesalamine/asacol, immunosuppression (6-MP, imuran), steroids, abx (rifaximine, cipro, or flagyl) for flares, rowasa enemas if colorectal dz, flagyl for anal dz, infliximab (remicade) if refractory to above or EC fistula/perianal disease; sx: if stricture, refractory to medical rx (ex. persistent SBO/bleeding/infection), fistula, perf, toxic megacolon; avoid sx x6 wks after flare, x12 wks if +remicade, minimize bowel resected, preserve ileocecal valve if possible, options include strictureplasty and SBR

Radiation proctitis – dx: 4500 rads → 1% incidence, 6500 rads → 50%; rx: steroid, carafate enemas → if persistent get bx to r/o ca and perform endoscopic intervention w/ Nd:YAG laser or ABC→ if continues consider diversion; emergent APR for uncontrollable bleeding; some pts may be candidates for rectal resection and coloanal pull through in elective setting

Radiation enteritis – dx: UGIS; rx: steroids (if acute), diet changes (low-residue) or TPN prn, cholestyramine and antimotility agents for diarrhea, SBR for strictures

Meckel's – dx: intraop finding or technetium (Meckel's) scan; rx: resect in all children, only symptomatic adults or adults in whom Meckel's flare may present diagnostic dilemma in future (ex. Crohn's)

Duodenal tumors – dx: EGD w/ biopsy, CTAP/CXR to stage if +adenocarcinoma; rx: adenoma → polypectomy if possible, local excision via duodenotomy vs Whipple if villous or otherwise unresectable; adenocarcinoma → Whipple

Peutz-Jeughers – SB hamartoma, mucocutaneous melanotic nodules, cancer (GI tract, pancreas, breast, lung, cervix, ovaries/testes), surgery for symptomatic lesions, asymptomatic polyp > 1.5 cm not amenable to endoscopic resection, or malignancy

LARGE BOWEL

Colonoscopy – average risk: 50 yrs, annual DRE + fecal occult blood testing/flex sig q5yrs or colonoscopy q5-10 yrs; moderate risk = pt with personal hx or first degree relative with neoplasia, start at 40 yrs or 10 yrs prior to cancer incidence, colonoscopy q5 yrs; if adenomatous polyp, colonoscopy q1yr until negative; high risk – annual colonoscopy + genetic screening for family prn for FAP (start age 12), HNPCC (start 5 yrs younger than youngest fam member w/ CRC), IBD > 10 yrs duration; if FAP also need EGD to screen duodenum for ca and CTAP for desmoid tumors. HNPCC = 3 relatives, 2 generations, 1 pt w/ CRC at age < 50, not FAP.

Polyps – carcinoma-in-situ = confined to mucosa → polypectomy adequate; malignant polyp = into submucosa = T1 cancer, polypectomy alone OK if completely excised, not poorly differentiated, no lymphovascular invasion, margin negative. If any of the above not true → proceed to colonic resection

CRC staging – I: T1-2, II: T3-4, III: N1-N2; IV: M1; N1=1-3LNs, N2=4+LNs

Colon cancer – get 5 cm margins, obtain >12 LNs, adjuvant chemo FOLFOX x 6months if high risk stage II (T4, lymphovascular invasion, obstruction, T3 with local perf, close/positive margins) or stage III (+LNs)

Rectal cancer – can do transanal excision if T1N0 with favorable histology, < 8 cm from anal verge, well diff with no lymphovascular or perineural invasion, 1/3 circumference and < 3 cm in diameter (sx = 1 cm margin, full thickness), otherwise need radical resection; high T2N0 (ie. away from sphincter) → radical resection; low T2N0 (ie. near sphincter) or T3-T4 or N1 (Stage II/III) → neoadjuvant XRT/chemo with FOLFOX/4500 rads x6 wks followed by radical resection; sx options: LAR if can achieve >2 cm distal margin, APR if LAR not possible or if tumor invades levators/sphincter; if T1-T2N0 no adjuvant, if T3+, N1+ then give adjuvant chemo x6 mo (options = 5-FU/LV, FOLFOX, capecitabine +/- oxaliplatin).

CRC follow up - hx/PE/CEA q3 months for 2 years, then q6 mos for years 3-5; colonoscopy 1 yr after resection (or sooner if no complete colonoscopy was done), then q1-3 yrs; CTCAP in high risk pts or pts s/p metastatectomy

Cytoreductive surgery with HIPEC (heated intraperitoneal chemo) – applications: pseudomyxoma peritonei (mucinous cystadenoma of appendix), appendiceal ca with peritoneal involvement, CRC with low-volume peritoneal involvement

Cecal volvulus – rx: ileocecectomy w/ primary reanastomosis (stomas only if very worried)

Sigmoid volvulus – rx: colonoscopic detorsion w/ placement of rectal tube, same-admission bowel prep and sigmoidectomy

Ischemic colitis - dx: CTAP, sigmoidoscopy; rx: abx, NPO, IVF, optimize hemodynamics (CVP/swan/inotropes prn), serial exams, rescope if worsens clinically or on labs, OR if perf, gangrene on scope, clinical deterioration

Ulcerative colitis – indications for surgery: fulminant colitis, perf, refractory to meds, anemia, intolerable med side effects, LGD (20% ca risk), HGD (50% ca risk), cancer. Rx: if acute → total colectomy w/ end ileostomy, later completion proctectomy +/- IPAA, if elective → options: total proctocolectomy w/ end ileostomy, total proctocolectomy w/ IPAA, subtotal colectomy w/ ileorectal anastomosis (only if minimal rectal dz, need for continued surveillance of rectal stump)

LGIB – dx/rx: NPO/IV access/transfuse prn/foley/ICU, NG lavage to r/o UGI source, colonoscopy w/ intervention, angio w/ embo (IR may ask for bleeding scan first), if chronic bleed and not localized on EGD/colonoscopy get capsule study vs push/double-barrel enteroscopy to eval SB source; sx: OR if 4 units in 24h, 10 units total, persistent HD instability, bleeding refractory to non-operative rx; safest option = subtotal colectomy w/ end ileostomy, make sure check SB for possible source, can consider segmental colectomy, if well-localized on angio or scope

Ogilvie's – dx: r/o mechanical obstruction with CTAP or gastrografin enema, cecal diameter >12 cm more worrisome; rx: NPO, IVF, hold narcs, replete lytes, d/c anticholinergic meds, serial exam/AXR, if no improvement or >12 cm → neostigmine (1-2 mg IV, can repeat dose, need cardiac monitor x30' for potential bradycardia), cannot give if HR < 60, SBP < 90, 2nd-3rd degree heart block, bronchospasm, pregnancy, Cr >3, if fails or contraindicated → colonoscopy (leave in tube) → if fails OR for R hemicolectomy w/ end ileostomy + mucus fistula (cecostomy also option though high risk of local complications)

ANUS

Anal fissure – if anterior → w/u for HIV, syphilis, CD/UC, leukemia, TB, cancer; medical rx → fiber, stool softeners, sitz baths, local anesthetics, diltiazem or NTG cream; surgical rx → lateral internal sphincterotomy

Anal fistula - rx: fistulotomy if < 30% external sphincter involved anteriorly, < 50% posteriorly; if > then above →fistula plug or fibrin glue or staged fistulotomy (1st stage, cut from internal opening of fistula to dentate line, allow to heal before 2nd stage → cut remaining sphincter)

Condyloma acuminatum – rx: EUA, anoscopy, excision/cauterization with bx, postop=imiquimod, other options include podophyllin, cryotherapy, trichloroacetic acid (TCA)

Anal intraepithelial neoplasia = AIN = SCC in situ = Bowen's disease – rx: local excision if small/isolated/macroscopic; if wide give imiquimod and reevaluate; if invasive SCC → rx as below

Anal canal SCC – anal canal=upper border of anal sphincter (puborectalis/anorectal ring) to anal verge; dx: anoscopy w/ bx, colonoscopy, CTAP, examine inguinal LNs and get FNA if clinically positive → chemoradiation with 5-FU/mitomycin C/4500 rads, boost dose to groin if +inguinal LNs, evaluate 8-12 wks later → 1) if progression of disease then bx, restage, and do APR if no mets 2) if persistent disease, reevaluate again in 4 wks → if progression/no regression, restage and perform APR if no mets; if +regression, continue to follow exam q3-6 mo and restage/consider APR if disease fails to regress or progresses at any point ; perform superficial inguinal LND if persistently positive or inguinal recurrence; metastatic disease rx w/ 5-FU/cisplatin.

Anal margin SCC – anal margin=anal verge to 5-6 cm around it; if T1N0 lesion do WLE, re-excise if positive margins; otherwise treat like anal canal SCC

Anal BCC – WLE w/ clear margins

Intraepithelial adenocarcinoma of anus = Paget disease – need colonoscopy to r/o synchronous colon ca, rx=WLE w/1 cm margin and mapping biopsies, if invasive ca → rx as rectal cancer

Anal adenocarcinoma – rx as rectal adenocarcinoma

Anal melanoma – WLE if possible, APR if involves sphincter or pt incontinent; benefit of SLNBx/LND/chemo/XRT uncertain; very poor prognosis

Anorectal stricture – medical rx: stool softener, fiber, observation for 3-6 months; anal dilation; sx – if muscular stricture→ lateral internal sphincterotomy; if mucosal stricture, stricturotomy (divide longitudinally in 3-4 quadrants and leave wounds open), if above fail → advancement flap

Rectovaginal fistula - rectal or vaginal advancement flap are primary options; in radiation induced fistula → wait 6 months, if local tissues healthy do advancement flap; if fails, use interposition flap using non-radiated tissue (ex. gracilis) or rectal resection with coloanal anastomosis and omental interposition; if sphincter incompetent/pt incontinent also requires overlapping sphincteroplasty; malignant fistula → diversion, neoadjuvant therapy, possible pelvic exenteration

Pilonidal disease – abscess → incision off midline + drainage, shave area, sitz baths, abx prn for DM/cellulitis/immunocompromised; definitive sx → unroofing or sinus excision

Anal incontinence – dx: anal manometry, anal USG, pudendal nerve testing; rx: bulking agents observation x6 months, plication sphincteroplasty if problem persists and abnormal test(s) noted above

Rectal prolapse – dx: colonoscopy, rectal manometry, transit study (markers pass by 5d) to r/o colonic inertia; rx: rectopexy vs rectopexy/resection (if redundant or constipation), Altemeier procedure if high risk

Hemorrhoids –dx: staging (applies to internal only) - I = no prolapse, II = prolapse w/ spontaneous reduction, III = prolapse w/ manual reduction, IV = prolapse, irreducible; rx: stage I/II/early III internal → rubber band ligation vs sclerotherapy (cottonseed oil, ethanolamine), stage III/IV internal→ hemorrhoidectomy; external → excise if +thrombosis and <24 hrs

Solitary rectal ulcer syndrome (SRUS) – dx: may be due to rectal intussusception and outlet obstruction, bx to r/o ca; rx = medical (increased fiber/fluid), carafate enemas, biofeedback; rx: surgery for severe symptoms (ex. rectal prolapse, bleeding requiring transfusion) → sigmoid resection w/ rectopexy; colostomy is option of last resort

HEPATOBILIARY

Liver mass eval - hx: hepatitis, cirrhosis, previous cancer, OCP use; dx: CTAP → MRI if diagnosis still in question →if still unsure get tagged rbc scan to r/o hemangioma, colloid scan to r/o FNH → bx rarely indicated, only if above studies not diagnostic; labs: tumor markers (AFP → elevated in HCC; CEA → elevated in metastatic colon ca), hepatitis panel, LFTs, INR, Cr.

Liver simple cyst – dx: make sure no papillary projections/daughter cysts/calcification/septation on imaging; if symptomatic → laparoscopic fenestration, if not surgical candidate → aspiration and injection (doxy, tetracycline, etoh, hypertonic saline), CANNOT do this if +bile on aspiration

Polycystic liver disease – sx if symptomatic; if limited # of large, accessible cysts → lap fenestration, if diffuse involvement → resection and possible fenestration of selected cysts, if little intervening normal parenchyma → OLT

Liver cystadenoma – dx: mural nodularity or papillary projections, multilocular; rx = surgery - enucleation (if no evidence of malignancy), resection (if suspected malignancy/deep lesions/biliary communication)

Echinococcal cyst – dx: daughter cysts; rx: preop/postop albendazole, if medically unfit → aspiration/injection of hypertonic saline followed by reaspiration, if medically fit can do cystectomy (first aspirate and inject w/ hypertonic NaCL in OR if thin walled b/c of risk of spillage) or liver resection (favor if multilocular, destruction of liver, proximity to major structures); if you do cystectomy and find that communication with duct exists → primary closure if < 5 mm size, CBD T tube or RYHJ or conversion to hepatic resection if > 5 mm

Hemangioma – dx: CTAP (peripheral retention of contrast @ venous phase), get +tagged rbc scan if CT/MRI non diagnostic; rx: enucleate if symptomatic/grows; may cause Kasabach-Merritt syndrome (consumptive coagulopathy with thrombocytopenia)

Focal nodular hyperplasia (FNH) – dx: CTAP (stellate scar), get +colloid scan if CT/MRI nondiagnostic; rx – resection if symptomatic

Hepatic adenoma – dx: CTAP (heterogeneity, hypervascular with contrast); rx: discontinue OCP, if < 4 cm + asymptomatic observe with serial imaging/AFP, if > 4 cm or grows or pt desires pregnancy or symptomatic → resection; if ruptured → embolization followed by elective resection

HCC – dx: suspect if growing nodule/elevated AFP in cirrhotic liver, CTAP (homogeneous enhancement); rx – if preserved liver function → resection if single lesion < 5 cm; if impaired liver function → OLT if fulfills Milan criteria (single lesion< 5 cm, three lesions each < 3 cm); RFA/TACE/sorafenib(tyrosine kinase inhibitor) if not candidates for either resection or OLT

Hepatic abscess – dx: entamoeba serology, CTAP (also serves to r/o other intraabdominal infxn causing secondary abscess); rx: if pyogenic → abx (broad spectrum) and perc drainage; if amebic → abx only (flagyl), reserve drainage for refractory abscess; if fungal change abx to caspo/micafungin; if concomitant source needs sx or mult abscesses or contraindication to perc drain (ex. ascites, coagulopathic) → surgery, remember to BIOPSY wall

Portal hypertension (varices) – prevention: propranolol; rx: endoscopy w/ banding, octreotide, vasopressin → TIPS if continued/recurrent bleeding → if bleeds after TIPS check patency w/ USG, consider redo TIPS; progressive liver disease → OLT; role of surgical shunts: extrahepatic causes of portal HTN (schistosomiasis, Budd-Chiari), compliance issues making TIPS poor option (need surveillance USG to follow shunt), TIPS failure, last ditch option in bleeding pt

Types of shunts – total: side-to-side portacaval, end-to-side portocaval or mesocaval interposition w/ 10 mm wide shunt; partial: 8 mm mesocaval shunt, splenorenal shunt

Refractory ascites – diuretics, large-volume paracentesis, TIPS, peritoneovenous shunting, portosystemic shunting, OLT eval

Hepatic encephalopathy – evaluate for GI bleeding and SBP; rx: address underlying/exacerbating cause prn, lactulose, protein restriction, rifaximine

Budd-chiari syndrome – dx: USG w/doppler, CTAP or MRI, get hypercoagulability workup; rx: anticoagulation, sodium restriction, diuresis, but high mortality rate (90% in 2 yrs) if medical rx only. So refer for OLT if possible, if no OLT possible → 1) PV totally occluded → mesocaval shunt; 2) PV partially occluded → TIPS; 3) PV not occluded → TIPS unless acute, then may consider thrombolysis/angioplasty/stent followed by TIPS

Biliary injury/bile leak – stabilize pt, treat sepsis w/ abx prn, drain biloma if present, ERCP, PTC if proximal obstruction, consider temporary biliary stent if injury is amenable, and go to OR for delayed reconstruction w/ RYHJ

Mirizzi syndrome – gallstone impacted @ junction of cystic duct w/ CBD causes erosion of CHD and obstruction (elevated transaminases/bilirubin); if small CHD → chole and primary closure; if large defect → chole and RYHJ

Choledochal cysts – type I=fusiform → excise, RYHJ; type II=diverticular → excise, primary closure + T tube; type III=intraduodenal → kocher, duodenotomy, identify CBD/PD, resect, sphincteroplasty; type IVa =intrahepatic + extrahepatic cysts → if unilateral intrahepatic then lobectomy w/ excision of extrahepatic biliary tree/RYHJ, if bilateral intrahepatic then bilateral stents of intrahepatic biliary tree w/ excision of extrahepatic biliary tree/RYHJ; type IVb =mult extrahepatic cysts → resection w/ RYHJ; type V=Caroli disease → 1) if unilateral + no cirrhosis do lobectomy with RYHJ, 2) if bilateral + no cirrhosis medical rx with abx, biliary drainage, ursodiol, 3) if cirrhosis, or if above options fail refer for OLT

Primary sclerosing cholangitis (PSC) – dx: 90% have UC (conversely 5% UC have PSC), 15-20% will develop cholangiocarcinoma, get liver bx to dx PSC only if ERCP findings not conclusive (ie. in "small duct" disease); rx: treat symptoms (cholestyramine, antihistamines, abx if infection), if dominant stricture r/o malignancy with ERCP brushing cytology and EUS-FNA, and perform dilation → if dilation fails or suspected CCA → excision with RYHJ; if cirrhosis refer for OLT

Cholangiocarcinoma – 1) intrahepatic → resection or if unresectable then gemcitabine/cisplatin, TACE, RFA, XRT; 2) extrahepatic → Whipple if behind/in pancreas, duct excision/ portal lymphadenectomy if above pancreas, if unresectable place stent; 3) Klatskin → tissue dx unnecessary, if no extension or unilateral involvement of portal structures, resect extrahepatic bile duct w/ portal lymphadenectomy, if prox margin of hepatic duct positive or lobe/PV involved→ add lobar resection, if distal margin of CBD positive → add Whipple; 4) unresectable/met disease → gemcitabine, cisplatin, XRT, stent/drain prn

Gallbladder cancer – stage I (T1N0) → simple chole suffices, if cystic duct margin + then CBD excision with RYHJ; stage II (T2N0) or stage III (T3N0 or any T, N1)→ radical chole = chole + liver resection (IVB/V) + portal lymphadenectomy (some also do CBD excision); stage IV resectable (T4N0M0 or T4N1M0) → as above for stage II/III, but may need formal hepatic lobectomy; stage IV unresectable (M1 or any T, N2 – distant nodes positive)→ palliation +/- experimental rx, existing chemo/XRT not effective.

Gallstone ileus – dx: pneumobilia on AXR, CTAP; rx: run entire small bowel to locate all stones, make longitudinal incision proximal to stone, milk back, close transversely, SBR if necrosis/perf, safe option = leave fistula alone but if stable/low risk/young → can also consider cholecystectomy/takedown of fistula

PANCREAS

Acute pancreatitis – dx = USG to r/o gallstones, CTAP if severe/worsens, follow symptoms/exam/amylase/lipase/LFTs; rx: NPO, IVF, ICU prn, pain control, TPN or post-ampullary TF, DVT/stress ulcer prophylaxis, early ERCP if bilis rising, FNA if concern for infected necrosis, necrosectomy if +infection, chole once pain-free if mild/moderate pancreatitis (ERCP w/ sphincterotomy if not operative candidate), delay chole after discharge if severe pancreatitis. Ranson criteria: on admission - age >55, wbc>16, gluc>200, AST >250, LDH>350; at 48 hrs - hct fall >10, BUN inc >5, Ca<8, PaO2<60, base deficit>4, fluid sequestration>6L: if score is 5-6 → 40% mortality. If score is 7-8 → 100% mortality

Pancreas divisum – dx: ERCP, secretin stim (EUS or MRCP) – if duct dilation persists then higher likelihood of improvement w/ intervention, MRCP or CTAP to eval parenchyma; rx: options = ERCP with sphincterotomy or stent insertion vs surgical sphincteroplasty of accessory papilla; if repeat symptoms with stenosis s/p sphincteroplasty → consider pancreatic head resection

Chronic pancreatitis – rx=chole if +gallstones, EtOH cessation, DM control, panc enzymes, analgesics, perc etoh ablation, ERCP w/ stent or sphincterotomy and stone removal; sx: consider if fails medical rx 1) if dilated PD only → Puestow, 2) if dilated PD + HOP dz → duodenum-preserving resection of pancreatic head + RYPJ (Beger – RYPJ to tail of pancreas, Frey – longitudinal RYPJ), 3) if normal PD + HOP dz → whipple, 4) if normal PD + body/tail dz → distal panc

Pancreatic ca – dx: consider preop biliary stent for: cholangitis, intractable pruritis, major nutritional deficiency; CTAP or MRCP, CA19-9 level, get EUS-FNA bx and give neoadjuvant chemoXRT if borderline resectable (borderline = SMV/PV contact or encasement without long-segment occlusion, GDA +/- short segment hepatic artery encasement, <180 deg abutment of SMA; unresectable = mets, long-segment SMV/PV occlusion, significant encasement of hepatic artery, >180 deg abutment of SMA, any abutment of celiac artery, aortic invasion, +LNs outside field of resection); rx: if no mets/resectable → sx; palliative rx=GI stent prn, biliary stent prn, if in OR already and find unresectable → biliary and enteric bypasses, EtOH injection to celiac plexus; best predictor of long-term survival=LN status; consider adjuvant chemo for all stages post-resection=gemcitabine or 5-FU/LV; follow w/ H&P/CTAP/CA19-9

Work-up of pancreatic cystic neoplasm – MRCP or CTAP, ERCP, EUS-FNA (send fluid for cytology, mucin, CEA, Ca 19-9, amylase)

Pancreatic pseudocyst – cyst fluid w/ high amylase level, low CEA/CA19-9; rx: observe w/ serial imaging, intervene if >6cm or symptomatic →ERCP to see if communicates, if not → can aspirate or place drain, if yes → endoscopic drainage (into stomach) or surgery (wait at least 6 wks from acute episode to allow wall to mature), remember to BIOPSY wall; if infected or unstable → external drainage only

Serous cystadenoma – benign, dx: cyst fluid w/low mucin/CEA, ERCP shows no connection w PD; rx=observe, sx if symptomatic or growth

Mucinous cystadenoma – malignant potential, dx: cyst fluid w/ high mucin/CEA>200, ERCP shows no connection w PD; rx=surgery

Solid pseudopapillary tumor – young pts, malignant potential, dx: "cystic"-appearing necrosis CTAP, FNA unhelpful; rx=surgery

Lymphoepithelial cyst – cyst fluid w/elevated CEA/Ca 19-9, NO mucin, cytology +squamous cells/lymphocytes/cholesterol; rx=observation, surgery if symptomatic

Autoimmune pancreatitis – causes mass effect in pancreas that can mimic ca, PD rarely dilated (as opposed to chronic pancreatitis), dx=IgG4 serology, FNA unhelpful; rx=steroids, repeat CT scan, if no improvement consider malignancy and diagnostic resection

Pancreatic lymphoma – local lymphadenopathy, LDH elevated, FNA helpful, rx=CHOP

Metastases to pancreas – renal cell carcinoma most common → rx=surgery if isolated dz

IPMN – key feature is connection with PD on ERCP, fluid analysis → high mucin, CEA variable; if main duct IPMN → surgery; if branch duct IPMN → surgery if symptomatic, cyst fluid w/CEA > 1000, CA 19-9 rising or >100, cyst size > 3 cm, mural nodules/thickened septum/associated mass/stricture, +family hx; sx: resect, send frozen section, if margin shows 1) cancer or HGD → re-resection 2) LGD → re-resection on case-by-case basis 3) negative → done. If observing branch-duct IPMN → annual Hx/PE/CA 19-9, MRCP vs CTAP, EUS + FNA w/ fluid analysis if IPMN enlarges/changes

Insulinoma – hx: eval for liver disease/etoh abuse (can also cause hypoglycemia), MEN-1 (**p**arathyroid, **p**ituitary, **p**ancreatic), dx: 72 hr fasting test (symptomatic hypoglycemia with elevated insulin, resolution with glucose, check c-peptide also), progression of localization studies = CT →MRI → EUS → arteriogram → portal vein sampling (octreotide scan usually not helpful); preop rx=octreotide or diazoxide; rx=sx, do IOUS or venous assays if no preop localization, enucleation if possible, whipple if deep/involves PD, debulk prn, if can't find tumor or don't have access to venous assays → distal panc (if still no tumor then refer to endocrine specialist, ? re-resection of pancreas); do subtotal pancreatectomy if MEN-1 (high rate of islet cell hyperplasia)

Pancreatic polypeptide secreting tumor – no symptoms, dx=PP level > 300

VIPoma – WDHA (watery diarrhea, hypokalemia, achlorhydria) syndrome, dx=VIP > 500, diarrhea when NPO; preop=octreotide, fluid resuscitation

Somatostatinoma – steatorrhea, gallstones, DM, dx=somastatin level

Glucagonoma – necrolytic migratory erythema (perioral, pretibial, intertriginous), wt loss, DM, DVT; dx=glucagon >500, low plasma amino acids, localize as in insulinoma; preop=TPN, insulin, correction of hypoaminoacidemia, octreotide; postop=octreotide

Pancreatic ascites- NPO, TPN, somatostatin, paracentesis, ERCP w/ stent, pancreatic resection if stent fails

SPLEEN/HERNIA

Overwhelming post splenectomy sepsis (OPSI) – s/p trauma → 0.5-1%, s/p malignancy → 2%, if peds splenectomy give prophylactic standing penicillin until age 18

Accessory spleen – dx: CT scan, technetium-labelled rbc or colloid scan

ITP – IVIG, prednisone, surgery if prolonged thrombocytopenia, severe thrombocytopenia, relapse or failure of medical therapy, prohibitive side effects, response rate = 75%

TTP –plasmapheresis, FFP 1st line; splenectomy for frequent relapses, response rate = 40%

Autoimmune hemolytic anemia – warm: steroids, if no remission or need high dose steroids → splenectomy, response rate = 70%; cold: avoiding cold, alkylating agents (chlorambucil/cyclophosphamide), plasmapheresis, NO steroids, NO splenectomy (erythrocytes are destroyed in liver)

Felty syndrome = rheumatoid arthritis, neutropenia, splenomegaly; rx = methotrexate/antirheumatics, G-CSF, splenectomy for failure of medical therapy, response rate=80%

Sarcoidosis – splenectomy for symptomatic splenomegaly, intractable pain, possible neoplasm

Hereditary spherocytosis – splenectomy + cholecystectomy (wait until >5 yrs old to decrease risk of OPSI)

Hereditary elliptocytosis – splenectomy if severe form of hemolysis

Sickle-cell anemia – splenectomy for splenic abscess or sequestration (but spleen usually autoinfarcts)

Hairy-cell leukemia – splenectomy rare, reserved for pancytopenia refractory to purine analogues

CML/CLL/thalassemia/myelofibrosis with myeloid metaplasia – splenectomy for severe symptoms (thrombocytopenia, splenomegaly)

Splenic cysts – sx if symptomatic, if asymptomatic simple cyst > 5 cm (rupture risk), or if echinococcal; operative options=splenectomy (multiple cysts, polycystic spleen, large central/hilar lesions, safest option for echinococcal cyst), fenestration/cystectomy (increased recurrence risk), partial splenectomy (polar lesions)

Lumbar hernia – Grynfeltt (superior) – borders = 12th rib, quadratus lumborum, internal oblique; Petit (inferior) - borders = iliac crest, lat dorsi, external oblique; rx=open or lap hernia repair w/ mesh

Obturator hernia – Howship-Romberg sign (hip/thigh pain w/ external rotation and hip extension), typical pt=old, female, rx=reduce hernia, incise obturator membrane prn to release, primary repair if small, mesh repair if large and no contamination, SBR prn

ADRENAL

Adrenal nodules (diagnosis) - evaluate for 1) hypercortisolism – if low dose (1 mg) dexamethasone suppression test does not suppress cortisol to <5, then check 24h urinary cortisol, if low no hypercortisolism, if high then +hypercortisolism. To figure out cause, 1st check ACTH → if ACTH low, then adrenal Cushing's, if ACTH high, then check high dose (8 mg) dexamethasone suppression test → +cortisol suppression implies pituitary source (get brain MRI), failure to suppress implies ectopic source (ex. paraneoplastic syndrome from other ca, get CTCAP) 2) hyperaldosteronism – suspect if hypokalemic and +HTN, if plasma aldosterone: renin ratio > 30, check 24h urine aldosterone under Na load conditions to confirm 3) pheochromocytoma – check serum metanephrines/normetanephrines, if equivocal check 24h urine metanephrines/catecholamines/VMA. If still unsure can perform clonidine suppression test (will not suppress in pheo; measure catecholamines after 0.3 mg po, if < 500 pg/cc no pheo).

Adrenal nodules (treatment) - resect if symptomatic/hormone-producing any size, or asymptomatic if >4 cm. If observing, check annual CT scan, annual screen for hypercortisolism, hyperaldosteronism, pheo. If grows > 1 cm, resect. If stable for 3 yrs, stop following.

Adrenal hypercortisolism – preop prep w/ ketoconazole prn, periop rx w/ corticosteroids; if unresectable of metastatic disease → mitotane or metyrapone

Aldosteronoma (Conn's syndrome) – preop prep w/ spironolactone/K/antihypertensives, localize w/ CTAP, SVS, NP-59 iodocholesterol scan; if cannot localize get captopril suppression test to r/o adrenal hyperplasia (will suppress in hyperplasia, but not for aldosteronoma). If hyperplasia → med rx only

Pheochromocytoma – r/o MEN-2 by hx/fam hx/Ca level/calcitonin level, localization progression: CTAP → MRI → I-131 MIBG → portosplenic vein testing; preop prep w/ phenoxybenzamine (10 mg qd, increase to 10 mg tid or until orthostatic/nasal congestion), add beta-blockers if tachy or symptomatic; sx: a-line, drips available for rx of HTN/hypotension, do adrenalectomy, IOUS prn, debulk prn, can give glucagon after resection to check for occult tumor – will inc BP/HR; if metastatic/unresectable, then debulk or use radioactive 131-I MIBG/chemotherapy; f/u: urinary studies q3mo, then q1yr; if +MEN, also eval family members

Adrenocortical carcinoma – dx: suspect if large adrenal mass, CTAP may show heterogeneity/irregular margins/hemorrhage/local invasion, also get CT chest to stage if likely cancer; sx: en bloc resection if no mets/physically feasible; XRT for incomplete resection, advanced local disease, aggressive tumors; mets → cisplatin; rx for hypercortisolism → mitotane (need adrenal replacement therapy if on this med - can also be used in pts with Cushing's syndrome 2/2 adrenal adenoma if non-operative)

Virilizing tumors - check serum DHEA/testosterone, urinary 17 ketosteroids/7 hydroxysteroids

Feminizing tumors – check estrogen (will be high) and FSH/LH (will be low), r/o testicular tumor

Adrenal metastasis – if suspect met, 1st r/o hormone-producing tumors (most importantly pheo), then get FNA bx (this is the rare instance in which you consider bx of an adrenal mass); rx = adrenalectomy if resectable/no other mets, primary controlled, favorable path (see rx pulm mets)

SKIN/SOFT TISSUE

BCC – low risk → 5 mm margin (trunk/extremities < 2 cm diameter lesion, head/neck < 1 cm lesion, sensitive area – eyes, ears, nose, moth, hands, feet < 6 mm, not recurrent, not immunocompromised, no perineural invasion); high risk→ if does not meet above criteria, get 1 cm margin

SCC – low risk → 5 mm margin; high risk → 1 cm margin (similar criteria to BCC). XRT postop if + margin, neurovascular invasion, medial canthus eye/nose. Alternatives: cryo, topical chemo (5% 5-FU cream, 5% imiquimod for superficial BCC/actinic keratosis), XRT

Merkel cell carcinoma – 2 cm margin, obtain SLNBx, completion LND prn, adjuvant XRT, rx mets w/ cisplatin and etoposide

Dermatofibroma protuberans – 3 cm margin, XRT for close (<1 cm) or positive margins

Kaposi sarcoma – bx to exclude bacillary angiomatosis (similar appearance); rx=optimize HIV treatment, intralesional vinblastine or XRT for localized disease, doxorubicin for systemic disease

Angiosarcoma – 2 cm margin, adjuvant XRT, consider induction chemo (paclitaxel or doxorubicin) if would facilitate complete resection/potentially spare vital structures

Melanoma – staging: LDH/CXR/LFTs, PET/CTAP if palpable LNs, brain MRI if symptomatic or stage IV; rx: 0.5 cm margin if in-situ, 1 cm margin if < 1 mm thick, 2 cm margin if >1 mm thick or ulceration; SLNBx if > 1 mm thick (or <1 mm with ulceration), get complete regional LND INSTEAD of SLNBx initially if palpable node or primary over LN basin. If SLNBx positive then perform completion LND: 1) face – MRND, also superficial parotidectomy if tracer localizes there or SLNBx positive and primary is located in upper face (ie tumor would cross parotid on way to cervical SLN); 2) arms - ALND levels I-III (unlike breast which is only I-II); 3) legs - superficial inguinal LND, reserve deep inguinal LND for +Cloquet's node (most superior node in superficial LND), +deep LNs on CTAP, >= 4 positive nodes on superficial inguinal LND, but NOT if aortic lymphadenopathy on CT scan (would add comorbidity w/ no benefit); 4) trunk – get lymphoscintigraphy to determine draining nodal region(s), do SLNBx, perform completion LND in corresponding locations prn.
Satellite lesions (<2 cm from primary) – surgery with negative margin (no need for wide margin), XRT, consider referral for hyperthermic isolated limb perfusion with melphalan if unresectable, chemo if none of the above are options (cisplatin, IFN, IL-2); adjuvant rx for locoregional (satellite/in-transit/nodal mets) or > 4 mm thick primary → IFN (induction IV x1 month, SQ x11 months).

Soft tissue sarcoma – dx: core bx, excisional (if lesion <3 cm) or incisional bx if core non-diagnostic (orient bx scar longitudinally b/c you need to excise it at time of definitive resection); staging: T1<5 cm, T2> 5 cm; G = grade, runs 1-3, higher is worse; stage I = all G1 (assuming N0), stage II = all G2 or T1G3 (assuming N0), stage III – T2G3 or any N1, stage IV – M1; rx: resect, otherwise give neoadjuvant chemoXRT and reassess; 2 cm margin (although 1 mm margin is ok w/ fascia/nerves/arteries/bone), usually give adjuvant XRT (unless small < 5 cm, superficial, low grade, and wide margins obtained), consider doxorubicin-based chemo if large or high-grade; mets: doxorubicin-based chemo

RP sarcoma – dx: CTCAP or MRI, only need bx if considering neoadjuvant or if another dx is possible; rx: if unresectable, consider giving chemo/XRT and reassessing; if resectable, en-bloc resection w/ adjacent involved organs (make sure to prep colon also), give postop XRT if high grade, large, close margins, R1 resection.

VASCULAR
AAA – repair if symptomatic, dissection present also, >5.5 cm men, >5 cm women, growth > 1 cm/year or 0.5 cm/6 months, lower size criteria for Marfan's/Loeys-Dietz

Ruptured AAA – USG in ER (usually too unstable to get CTAP)

EndoAAA – EVAR-I/DREAM decreased short-term complications/mortality, no difference in cumulative survival compared to open; need angulation < 60 degrees, at least 15 mm non-aneurysmal fixation site proximally, at least 7 mm femoral artery diameter; postop: surveillance CTA @ 1,6, 12 months; endoleaks: I – prox/dist attachment site (endo repair, convert to open if no success), II – backflow (coil embo if aneurysm expanding), III – fabric tear/between graft components (endo repair), IV – graft porosity (no repair), V – endotension (exclude endoleak → if present, endo repair)

Thoracoabdominal aortic aneurysms – repair if symptomatic, >5.5 cm, >1 cm/year growth, dissection, lower size criteria for Marfan's/Loeys-Dietz; sx – paraplegia risk, so avoid periop hypotension and consider CSF drainage (maintain pressure 8-10 mm Hg during OR, 10-12 early postop, 12-15 after legs move); Crawford classification = I – near subclavian to above renals, II – near subclavian to below renals (highest risk for paraplegia), III – mid DTA to below renals, IV – distal DTA to below renals; exposure = thoracoabdominal incision, may need to divide diaphragm: type I-II → enter 6th ICS, III → 7th or 8th ICS, IV → 9th ICS

Carotid stenosis – CEA if symptomatic 50-99% (NASCET), asymptomatic 80-99% (safer threshold for board purposes, though ACAS suggests 60-99%); recurrent carotid stenosis – refer for carotid artery stenting if possible, if not available then redo CEA (same criteria as above), may need patch angioplasty if recurrence is due to myointimal hyperplasia (interposition graft if patch angio not possible)

Carotid artery aneurysm – angiogram first with trial occlusion with balloon (heparinize, inflate balloon 30 seconds, observe for symptoms, usually backpressures > 70 mm Hg OK) – rx: 1) not extending to skull base → excision + graft 2) extending to skull base and does not tolerate trial occlusion → external-carotid to internal-carotid bypass (Neurosurg) and ligation, followed by anticoagulation, 3) extending to skull base and DOES tolerate trial occlusion → ligation, followed by anticoagulation. Possible endovascular rx also

Vertebral artery aneurysm - >80% resolve spontaneously, manage non-op with anticoagulation

Upper extremity arterial occlusive disease – DBI (digital brachial index), MRA/CTA/angio, rx=cold avoidance, tobacco abstinence, Ca channel blockers, corticosteroids, immunosuppression if vasculitis (ex. temporal arteritis, Takayasu, giant cell arteritis), avoid revascularization in "inflammatory phase"; sx=endovascular rx (short segment) vs open revascularization (long segment); open options: subclavian transposition (move subclavian to ipsilateral common carotid artery via transverse cervical incision) or carotid-subclavian bypass w/ graft

Steal syndrome s/p AVF – dx: compress fistula and check hand to see if improves, USG (will see reversed flow through artery distal to AVF), consider angio to check for anatomic issues; rx options = 1) ligation (use only if limb threatened or other options not effective) 2) banding (use if high flow through AVF) 3) DRIL procedure (use if low or normal flow through AVF) – ligate artery distal to arterial anastomosis of AVF, place vein graft from artery at least 5 cm prox to AVF to distal artery to bypass ligated section

TASC guidelines – type A - short segment → endovascular intervention may be attempted; type B/C – intermediate complexity → endovascular vs open; type D – long-segment occlusions → open option usually preferred. Endovascular intervention below knee → low success rate

Profundaplasty – profunda=posterolateral to CFA; pts may benefit from profundaplasty when undergoing lower extremity revascularization; options include - patch angioplasty vs endarterectomy/patch angioplasty vs angioplasty using hood of graft

Lower extremity peripheral vascular disease – dx: ABI, consider USG, get CTA vs MRA vs arteriogram (gold standard) once considering surgical intervention; medical rx: smoking cessation, exercise therapy, ASA, DM control, cholesterol reduction (LDL < 100), cilostazol (phosphodiesterase inhibitor, increases cAMP levels), pentoxifylline (reduces blood viscosity); surgery if claudication is lifestyle limiting and does not respond to medical rx, or progresses to limb-threatening ischemia (rest pain, gangrene, ulcers). Leriche syndrome = diminished femoral pulses, impotence, buttock claudication. Sx options in lower-extremity PVD: aortobifemoral bypass, axillofemoral bypass ("extraanatomic," redo, hostile abdomen, need to remove other infected graft/revascularize), iliofemoral bypass, fem-fem bypass, fem-pop bypass (above knee – prosthetic OK/below knee – vein much preferable), fem-distal bypass (low patency, vein much preferable), endovascular options (angioplasty, stent, atherectomy; better for iliofemoral dz vs infrapopliteal dz; avoid stenting across joint), goal = adequate inflow and outflow

Acute peripheral arterial emboli – rx: heparinize, consider initial angio from opposite side, usually expose femoral artery but may need to expose below-knee popliteal artery if need to do embolectomy on AT/PT/peroneal vessels), embolectomy in both directions (iliac: 4-6 Fr; femoropopliteal: 3-4 Fr; tibial vessels: 2-3 Fr), completion angio, fasciotomy prn (clinical suspicion for compartment syndrome, ischemia > 4hrs); postop rx: anticoagulation, rx reperfusion syndrome (hyperkalemia → rx prn, myoglobinuria → alkalinize urine/mannitol, acidosis → bicarb), eval w/ TTE and holter for cardiac source, CTCAP for aortic plaque if negative cardiac eval

Catheter-directed thrombolysis (CDT) – appropriate in pts with acute-on-chronic PVD, bypass better if recent imaging has shown long-segment stenosis/diffuse disease/limited runoff; rx: graft < 30 days old (early bypass failure) → graft revision, graft > 30 days but no viability threat → observation, graft > 30 days with threat to viability → CDT; sx: place catheter, d/c heparin, 5 mg TPA bolus followed by 0.25 to 0.5 mg/hr infusion, check coags/fibrinogen/cbc q4-6h, halve the rate if fibrinogen <150, stop infusion if < 100 (or give cryo); if limb improves → angio q12-24 hrs, if limb worsens → check catheter position and correct prn, consider open surgery

Popliteal/femoral artery aneurysm – main risk = thromboembolism, screen for other lower extremity and aortic aneurysm(s); rx – surgery if symptomatic, controversial if asymptomatic; sx – popliteal → distal/proximal ligation of aneurysm, interposition graft; femoral → excision and interposition graft

Pseudoaneurysm – rx: USG guided compression (if small), USG guided thrombin injection (if narrow neck), stent placement (temporizing measure, problematic if stent crosses joint), open repair (for symptomatic compression of vein/nerve, skin necrosis, large hematoma, failure of other methods).

Renal artery stenosis – treat if symptomatic (severe HTN, ischemic nephropathy, flash pulmonary edema) or asymptomatic if > 80%, > 60% in solitary kidney, rapidly progressive stenosis; rx: angioplasty (mid-distal renal artery, in-stent restenosis), angioplasty w/ stenting (ostial-proximal renal artery), aortorenal bypass; nephrectomy if kidney has <10% function and occluded artery

Acute mesenteric ischemia – rx: heparinize, embolectomy (embolus = distal to middle colic, thrombotic = origin of SMA), visceral artery bypass if acute-on-chronic, bowel resection w/ stoma/2nd look prn

Chronic mesenteric ischemia – rx: intervene if symptomatic and stenosis of at least 2 of 3 visceral vessels; sx: endovascular options (angioplasty/stent via upper extremity access – better angulation for catheter), surgical - bypass 1 or 2 arteries, inflow options = supraceliac aorta, infrarenal aorta, iliac artery, outflow = celiac, SMA (to get to SMA from supraceliac aorta, pass graft underneath pancreas)

AV fistula (AVF) – dx: check BP both arms, allen test if using radial, USG arteries, vein mapping (need at least 2-3 mm veins), USG deep veins to r/o DVT/stenosis; rx: place TDC at same time if need immediate access, use nondominant before dominant hand, use distal before proximal site, use vein before prosthetic; sx: radiocephalic (cimino) AVF, brachiocephalic AVF, basilic vein transposition AVF, AV graft, lower extremity AV graft; AVF needs 4-12 wks to mature, AV graft can be used within 10-14d

Venostasis disease – dx: USG to eval for DVT/perforators/valvular incompetence, ABI to r/o arterial disease; rx: local care, abx prn, leg elevation, compression therapy (unna boot – contains zinc + calamine, change q7d/compression stockings prn), skin grafting prn, GSV stripping/phlebectomy prn (NOT if +DVT), valve reflux sx for incompetent valves/SEPS prn for incompetent perforators

CRITICAL CARE

Hyperphosphatemia – rx: decrease phosphate intake, phosphate binders, HD prn

Hypercalcemia – rx: IVF, diuretics, bisphosphanates, steroids (esp for granulomatous dz), HD prn

Hyperkalemia – rx: make sure specimen not hemolyzed/contaminated with IVF, calcium gluconate if peaked T waves on EKG or significant hyperkalemia, kayexalate, d/c K/suspected meds, 10 units reg insulin/0.5 amp D50, bicarbonate, Lasix, HD prn

Hypermagnesemia – rx: elemental calcium, IVF, loop diuretics, HD prn

ARDS= $PaO2/Fio2 < 200$ with diffuse pulm infiltrates and no cardiac failure; ALI (acute lung injury)=$PaO2/Fio2$ 201-300; rx: increase PEEP, decrease tidal volume to 5-7 ml/kg, minimize FiO2, abx for PNA prn, HFOV if above fail, ECMO if possible reversibility

Sepsis –resuscitate (MAP>65, CVP 8-12, UOP >0.5 cc/kg/hr, Hgb target >10), abx, source control, vasopressors/inotropes prn, APC (xigris) if severe sepsis and no contraindication (bleeding risk), steroids/cort stim if possible adrenal insufficiency, glycemic control, VTE/stress ulcer prophylaxis, early nutrition

Cort stim – baseline should be > 25, cort stim with 250 mcg ACTH should produce cortisol levels >18-20 or +9 from baseline

Swan ganz – safe "normal or acceptable" values: cardiac index >= 2.2 L/min/m^2, SVR 800-1200 dynes, CVP < 12 mm Hg, PAD/PCWP < 15 mm Hg, RVSP < 30 mm Hg.

Cardiac failure/hypotension eval protocol – ABCs, PE, check UOP/place foley prn, IVF bolus, labs (including hct, cort stim if suspect adrenal insufficiency, troponin, CK-MB), CXR (chest tube prn PTX), EKG (ASA, beta-blocker, morphine, heparin gtt, NTG, cath prn MI), TTE (pericardial window prn effusion), a-line, CVP, Swan prn (nitric oxide start at 20 ppm, consider milrinone for pulm HTN/right heart failure), inotropes/IABP prn for CHF - low CI/high CVP/high PCWP (reasonable starting doses = epinephrine 0.02 mcg/kg/min, milrinone 50 mcg/kg load + 0.25-0.375 mcg/kg/min, dopamine 5 mcg/kg/min, dobutamine 5 mcg/kg/min), vasopressors prn (norepinephrine 1-8 mcg/min + titrate, vasopressin 0.04 units/min, phenylephrine 10 mcg/min + titrate)

Atrial fibrillation/flutter protocol – ABCs, EKG (can try adenosine 6 mg IV for dx if cannot tell from SVT or suspect reentrant tachycardia; if preop EKG shows delta wave → WPW → NO nodal blockers), PE (can try carotid massage if no bruit), labs (lytes – correct Mg, K), correct hypoxia, enzymes to r/o MI, if unstable → synchronized cardioversion starting w/ 100 J, if stable, medical rx → attempt to cardiovert w/ amiodarone gtt (bolus 150 mg, gtt 1 mg/min x6 hrs, then 0.5 mg/min x18 hrs, then change to amio 400 mg po q8h x 3 days, then 400 mg daily); rate control w/ metoprolol (IV 5 mg bolus x3 q15min prn, start PO also), diltiazem (0.25 mg/kg IV, can repeat in 15 min prn, gtt = 10 mg/min + titrate), digoxin (useful if hypotensive, load=1000 mcg in first 24 hrs, then start 250 mcg daily – less in CRI)

Respiratory failure/hypoxia eval protocol – ABCs, PE, labs w/ ABG, CXR, EKG, empiric diuresis if suspect pulmonary edema, ICU xfer, can try BIPAP if not ready to intubate, intubate prn, bronchoscopy, abx for PNA prn, chest tube prn, enteral nutrition, GI prophylaxis if intubated, CT chest w/ angio to r/o PE, TTE/CVP/swan if suspect cardiac etiology, can consider HFOV, ECMO if possible reversibility, trach in 7-10 days if no improvement,

Renal failure eval protocol - PE, labs, place/check/flush foley, labs, UA, urinary electrolytes (FENa - <1% prerenal, >1% ATN, but unreliable if +lasix), renal USG (esp if hydronephrosis/ureter injury possible), d/c nephrotoxic meds, renal dose other meds prn, d/c K, rx hyperkalemia prn, CVP prn, swan-ganz prn, diuretics prn to manage fluid overload, HD prn

Liver failure eval protocol – PE, labs (including hepatitis panel, INR, LFTs), liver USG with Doppler, supportive care = D10 for hypoglycemia, correct coags prn w/ FFP, rx hepatic encephalopathy (lactulose, neomycin), Child score includes **A**lbumin**B**ilirubin**C**oags + ascites + encephalopathy, MELD score includes bili/INR/Cr

Heparin – therapeutic dose = bolus 100 u/kg, then drip 15 u/kg/hr; therapeutic lovenox dosing = 1 mg/kg q12h (if normal Cr)

TPN – protein 1-1.5 g/kg/day, calories 25 kcal/kg/day, 50% non-protein calories as glucose and 50% free fatty acids, insulin prn, electrolytes (based on level), trace elements (zinc, selenium, copper, chromium); labs – glucose q6h, lytes/LFTs daily, prealbumin/lipid panel weekly

RCRI (revised cardiac risk index – Goldman) – high risk surgery (intraperitoneal, intrathoracic, suprainguinal vascular sx), CAD, CHF, CVA, DM, Cr >2 – if 2 or more risk factors out of 6 → beta blockade beneficial

PFTs – most important are FEV1 and DLCO – worry if either is < 40%

RSBI = rapid shallow breathing index = breaths per minute/tidal volume in L; if >100 → likely failure to wean vent/extubate (ie. 20 breaths per minute @ 600 ml TV is favorable, 40 bpm @ 300 ml is not)

ACLS - ABCs/IVF/labs in all, VT/VF – defibrillate (starting w/ 200 J), CPR, epi 1 mg IV q3-5 min OR vasopressin 40 units IV x1, give amiodarone 300 mg IV/Mg also if refractory to cardioversion, work up for myocardial ischemia, refer to EP for ICD placement; asystole – CPR, epinephrine 1 mg/atropine 1 mg q3-5 min, can attempt transcutaneous pacing; PEA – CPR, evaluate for underlying cause, epinephrine/atropine; symptomatic bradycardia – progression = atropine 0.5 mg → transcutaneous pacing → dopamine gtt → epinephrine gtt → transvenous pacing; hold nodal blocking agents, refer to EP for PPM placement.

PE/DVT – heparin gtt, follow plt count, TTE prn hypoperfusion/hypotension, IVC filter prn (indicated if PE burden significant or clinical status tenuous, contraindication to anticoagulation, repeat PE while on rx), if plts drop to < 100 or <50% of baseline eval for HIT, d/c heparin and start argatroban or hirudin gtt; if PE is submassive (RV dysfunction on TTE but HD stable) or massive (HD unstable) → place IVCF and consider IV TPA or suction embolectomy or surgical embolectomy (latter 2 options if expertise available and TPA contraindicated or fails)

Transfusion rxn – IVF, diuretics, direct Coombs (will be positive), hemolysis labs (LDH, hemoglobinuria, haptoglobin, bilirubin), repeat T+C w/ suspected unit of blood

TRAUMA

ABCD(disability= evaluate GCS)E(exposure)→ then proceed to secondary survey (FAST/c-spine XR/CXR/pelvicXR/foley/NGT prn/RUG prn/sigmoidoscopy prn/head to toe exam)

Airway control - ETT w/ direct laryngoscopy) → video laryngoscopy → fiberoptic bronch → surgical airway (use trach instead of cricothryoidotomy in peds, tracheal disruption, laryngeal fx)

ED thoracotomy - <15 min of CPR in penetrating trauma, not for blunt trauma (unless pericardial effusion suggesting tamponade)

Traumatic brain injury (TBI) - dx: CT head, GCS score 3-8=severe,9-12=moderate,13-15=minor; rx: drainage epidural hematoma prn, if severe TBI or deteriorating exam consider rescan/ICP monitor (maintain CPP > 60, ICP < 20) followed by stepwise rx of increased ICP prn: sedate/paralyze → drain CSF → controlled hyperventilation (pCO2 30-35) → mannitol/hypertonic saline → controlled hypothermia (33-35 degrees) / pentobarbital coma / craniectomy

Penetrating neck trauma – dx - don't forget CXR to r/o PTX, CT angio neck, EGD, bronchoscopy; hard signs=pulsatile/large hematoma, active bleeding, crepitus, hoarseness, dyspnea, large wounds, hematemesis, dysphagia; zone I – sternal notch to cricoid, zone II – cricoid to angle of mandible, zone III – above angle of mandible; rx - selective exploration of neck for all zones (OR for +hard signs or evidence of injury on studies), old school = exploration of ALL zone II injuries penetrating platysma

Thoracic trauma – dx: CXR, FAST, TTE if suspect cardiac injury/unexplained hypotension; rx: tube thoracostomy if hypotension and decr breath sounds, place also on opposite side if no hemodynamic response to first tube/resuscitation + pt too unstable to image, otherwise get CXR → chest tube prn; sx: thoracotomy if chest tube >1000 ml output initially, >200/hr, or large air leak (bronch also if +air leak). If FAST shows pericardial effusion: 1) stable/mild hypotension → OR for median sternotomy, intraop TEE to r/o valve injury/contusion 2) significant hypotension → can consider ER pericardiocentesis though OR for sternotomy preferred 3) in extremis → ER thoracotomy.

Transmediastinal GSW - if stable → after ABCs/eval will need bronch, barium swallow, CT angio, OR prn; if unstable → bilateral chest tubes, OR if does not respond or tube output high. If stabilizes get diagnostic w/u described above to r/o other injuries.

Rib fx/flail chest – intubate prn, pain control (consider epidural), pulmonary toilet, minimize fluid, monitor respiratory status closely given risk of pulm contusion

Blunt cardiac injury – dx - chest pain, EKG abnormalities (most common - sinus tach), troponin not that helpful; rx - observation if EKG abnormal / age >55 / cardiac hx, obtain TTE prn; OR for tamponade / valve injury / coronary injury, antiarrhythmics / inotropes / vasopressors prn, possible IABP / VAD

RP hematomas - in blunt trauma, explore all zone I and expanding zone II hematomas; in penetrating trauma, explore all zone I and II and III hematomas; exception (ie. avoid exploration) =stable retrohepatic hematoma

Diaphragmatic injury – suspect in L chest / upper abdominal penetrating injury (though can happen w/ blunt trauma also); dx/rx: if acute → laparoscopy for diagnosis (if no exlap done for other reasons), laparotomy for repair (may need to expose by mobilizing spleen / colon); if chronic → VATS / thoracotomy

Liver injury – if HD stable can manage nonoperatively, if +blush or falling hct → angio, if HD unstable or significant transfusion requirement (>4 units prbcs) or angio fails → OR; sx: pack, topical hemostatics, suture w/ blunt chromic needle, pringle, argon beam coagulator, if deep wound tract consider placing penrose tied around red rubber catheter and inflate "balloon" → temporary closure → 2nd look, if hepatic vein or retrocaval injury may need to isolate intrapericardial cava (requires sternotomy) and infrahepatic cava +/- atriocaval shunt, remember to place drain

Pancreas injury – explore ALL hematomas of pancreas if you are in OR already (mobilize panc w/ kocher and mattox maneuvers, evaluate for ductal injury, can give 1 mg secretin prn to help identify); if no exlap, perform ERCP; sx – place drain, tack omentum down, distal panc if transection or major injury to duct in neck / tail, Whipple only if totally destroyed yet stable (if borderline, Whipple in 2 stages – resect, then reconstruct at later date; if unstable, pack / drain and return once pt better)

Duodenal injury – if hematoma only (dx: GOO on CTAP w/ PO / NGT contrast or barium swallow) → NGT, TPN, observe for up to 3 wks, if persists do gastrojejunostomy; if injury in 2nd part, need to examine ampulla of vater and perform cholangiogram to determine if there is an injury to CBD; if in 3rd / 4th part, need to divide treitz to expose; sx=primary repair if possible, also place omental buttress / drain; if repair tenuous, consider diversion procedure – either pyloric exclusion with gastrojejunostomy or triple drainage (G tube, duodenostomy tube or retrograde J tube, feeding J tube); if defect too large, do roux-en-y duodenojejunostomy @ defect

Splenic injury – rx: any penetrating or blunt/HD unstable pt → safe answer = splenectomy, blunt/HD stable → observation, repeat CT scan 24-48 hrs, angio/embolization if pseudoaneurysm, OR if CT findings worse, significant transfusion requirement, becomes unstable

Renal injury – dx: OR if life-threatening bleeding, >50% devitalized parenchyma, UPJ avulsion, arterial thrombosis if both kidneys affected or pt only has single kidney; otherwise can proceed w/ nonoperative rx – strict bed rest until urine clears, repeat CT scan in 3-5 days in non-operative rx for grade IV/V injuries, if urinary leak persists place ureteral stents and drain urinoma, if cannot stent from below place perc nephrostomy tubes and eventual antegrade stents; if transfusion > 6 prbcs/hemodynamic changes → CT scan if stable, possible angio, OR (stable → salvage kidney if possible; unstable → nephrectomy)

Ureteral injury – contusion → stent/drain, and if severe resect/debride/reanastomose; ureteral injuries below iliac vessels → ureteroneocystostomy and psoas hitch prn; midureteral/upper ureteral injuries → ureteroureterostomy / UPJ repair over stent, less desirable option is transureteroureterostomy, large section loss may need conduit/interposition; if unstable → cutaneous ureterostomy or ligation of both ends followed by perc nephrostomy tube when stable, delayed reconstruction; later discovery of injuries (>2 wks) – prox diversion w/ perc nephrostomy tube, perc drainage of urinoma/abscess, antegrade stent placement across injured ureter, delayed (3 mo) reconstruction

Rectal injury – dx: rigid proctoscopy; rx: grades I + II (contusion/hematoma, laceration < 50% circumference) → repair if easily exposed + divert + presacral drain; grades III-V (laceration > 50% circumference, laceration extending to perineum) → resect/anastomosis/divert vs resect/Hartmann's, place presacral drain; if combined rectal/urinary injury, expose and repair/diverting stoma/suprapubic tube, drain, use omentum to isolate injuries

Abdominal compartment syndrome – dx: intraabdominal pressure > 20 mm Hg with new organ dysfunction (suspect if hypotension w/ high airway pressures, oliguria); rx: laparotomy; management of open abdomen – OR q48-72hrs, abx, vac dressing, diurese, close fascia superiorly and inferiorly gradually, if hernia remains you can 1) close skin primarily, if defect is small 2) biologic mesh, close skin over or vac 3) adaptic, vac alone, followed by STSG

Pelvic fracture – wrap w/ bed sheet if hypotensive in ED, if remains HD unstable and positive FAST → OR for exlap to address intraabdominal injuries then angio for pelvis then fixation prn, if HD unstable and negative FAST → angio then fixation prn, if HD stable → fixation prn. Assess for urethral/bladder and rectal injury if suspicion exists (blood @ urethral meatus/high riding prostate → RUG, possible cystogram; if gross blood on rectal exam → proctoscopy). If open perineal wound → will need diverting colostomy. If open groin wound → no diversion needed.

Vascular injury – dx: hard signs = pulsatile bleeding, expanding hematoma, thrill/bruit, ischemia → OR; soft signs = decreased ABI/pulses, fracture or projectile near major artery, nerve deficit, stable hematoma → consider duplex or angio; rx: shunt if necessary (can temporize during transport, damage-control sx, or fracture reduction); end-to-end or primary repair if possible, interposition w/ vein (preferable) or prosthetic prn; repair veins if possible, try especially hard NOT to ligate the suprahepatic IVC, portal vein, R renal vein (need nephrectomy if you do this - OK however to divide L renal vein b/c of collateral drainage via adrenal/gonadal veins); IVC injury – satinsky partial clamp if possible, prox/distal sponge sticks prn, if posterior wall injury → go through anterior wall to repair; fasciotomy prn (>4-6 hr ischemia, severe soft tissue injury, major venous injury/ligation, unreliable PE)

Normal extremity compartment pressure - 5-10 mm Hg; fasciotomy if 25-30+ or clinical suspicion or prophylactic (>4 hrs ischemia)

BURNS/THERMAL INJURY

Burn management – 1) ABC – laryngoscopy/bronch if airway injury, intubate prn, check carboxyhemoglobin (normal is <10%) → 100% o2 or hyperbaric if elevated 2) assess for other traumatic injuries 3) IVF - Parkland formula = 4 x weight in kg x % BSA burned, give ½ in first 8 hrs, ½ in next 16 hrs (count only 2nd degree burns or greater) 3) wounds – escharotomy prn if thoracic compartment syndrome ("shield" incisions) or extremity compartment syndromes, tetanus, topical abx, early wound excision/grafting of deep 2nd degree burns or greater, limit to 1-2 hrs OR time or 10-15% TBSA, 12/1000" thickness dermatome for STSG, scalpel for FTSG, systemic abx if infection (10x5 bacteria), use biobrane (silicone film) or allograft temporarily if infected and follow quantitative cx, eventually replace w/ autograft 4) GI – stress ulcer prophylaxis, nutrition (protein 3 mg/kg/day, higher for children, 25kcal/kg/day + 40 kcal x percentage burn) 5) pain management 6) DVT prophylaxis

Topical abx – bacitracin (superficial penetration); silvadene (superficial and intermediate penetration) – does not penetrate eschar, leukopenia; sulfamylon (intermediate and deep) – penetrates eschar, cartilage, causes pain/metabolic acidosis; silver nitrate (superficial and intermediate) – stains, hyponatremia

Hypothermia – ABC, utox, EKG/telemetry, remove wet clothing, cover w warm/dry blankets, heating pads, warm bath, heated IVF, invasive measures (ex. peritoneal lavage, ECMO) if severe hypothermia (<27 degrees Celsius)

Frostbite – correct systemic hypothermia, rewarm with bath (44 degrees Celsius), tetanus, pain control, ASA, dressing changes, debride clear blisters and apply aloe, leave hemorrhagic blisters intact, await demarcation

Electrical injury – ABC, eval and rx for burns and other traumatic injuries (ex. long bone/spinal fx from falls/tetany), monitor cardiac rhythm 24-72h, document neuro exam (can cause acute transient nervous system injury, delayed neuro syndromes also), document ocular exam (can cause cataracts), eval and rx for extremity compartment syndrome prn, evaluate and rx for myoglobinuria prn (alkalinize urine/IVF/mannitol)

Hydrofluoric acid – c/b hypocalcemia, monitor level closely, inject 10% calcium gluconate, may use intraarterial infusion

PEDIATRICS/UROLOGY

Esophageal atresia (EA)/tracheoesophageal fistula (TEF) – dx: CXR (NGT coils), if unclear give 1-2 ml barium to confirm, r/o renal/cardiac anomalies; types – A = EA only, B = EA + proximal TEF, C = EA + distal TEF (most common), D = EA + both prox and distal TEF, E = H type TEF; rx of types A-D: if pt intubated move ETT distal to TEF, NGT, elevate head of bed, abx if PNA, OR for primary repair unless PNA/ARDS/vented, low birth weight, congenital anomalies → then consider placing G tube, J tube, delayed repair; if long-gap atresia, may need serial bougienage via G tube or conduit (gastric, colon); rx type E – delayed presentation (PNA, failure to thrive, bronchospasm) → dx w/ esophagram/EGD → rx: division of fistula via cervical incision

Biliary atresia – dx: HIDA, USG, liver bx, check alphi-1 antitrypsin level (for deficiency) and sweat chloride test (for CF), hemolysis/hepatitis labs; rx: Kasai, actigall, fat soluble vitamins, OLT if failed Kasai/cirrhosis

Gastroschisis/omphalocele – dx: omphalocele = midline, covered w/ peritoneum, may contain liver, associated with other birth defects; gastroschisis = on R, no peritoneum, no other organs, no associated anomalies; rx: NGT, IVF, cover bowel, abx, if omphalocele assess for associated defects, sx = primary closure if possible, use silo and close gradually (may need TPN in this situation b/c of ileus)

Hypertrophic pyloric stenosis – abnormal dimensions of pylorus >= 3.5 mm thick (each wall), >= 15 mm long; NO NGT (worsens hypokalemic hypochloremic metabolic alkalosis); need to resuscitate and correct lytes before operating (give D51/2NS and add K once UOP OK); sx = pyloromyotomy

Meconium ileus – dx: AXR – soap bubble sign, if +calcifications → suggests complicated meconium ileus = bowel perforation/meconium peritonitis, get sweat chloride test for CF, barium enema if no perf (eval for microcolon, filling defects demonstrating meconium); rx: if no perf → NGT, IVF, abx, fluoro-guided water-soluble contrast enemas, if medical rx fails or +perf → OR, SBR prn, washout bowel, create double-barrel stomas to irrigate postop

Necrotizing enterocolitis (NEC) – dx: AXR = pneumatosis and/or portal venous gas; rx: NPO, TPN, resuscitate, abx, serial AXRs, OR if free air/clinically worsens, multiple stomas/2nd look prn

Duodenal atresia – dx: AXR = double bubble, UGIS if unsure, if Down's syndrome eval for heart defects; rx: duodenojejunostomy

Intestinal atresia – dx: UGIS, also do barium enema to r/o Hirschsprung's and confirm colon present/normal size; rx: resect atretic segment and anastomose

Intussusception – dx: USG (+target sign); rx: if perf/peritonitis → OR; if no perf/peritonitis → reduce w/ fluoro-guided barium enema, can repeat if recurs, if enema fails go to OR and reduce only (do not resect unless cannot reduce, obvious pathological lead point, or bowel not viable)

Malrotation – dx: UGIS (SB to R, colon to L); rx: Ladd's procedure

Congenital diaphragmatic hernia – dx: CXR; rx: stabilize respiratory status, HFOV/ECMO prn, then repair

Hirschsprung's disease – dx: barium enema (dilated segment has ganglia, narrow segment does not), rectal bx; rx: colostomy @ dilated colon (bx to make sure +ganglions), delayed pull-through procedure

Imperforate anus – dx: lateral pelvic radiography (wait 24h for pouch dilation, place marker @ anal dimple, if < 1 cm distance then primary repair, if > 1 cm distance then colostomy/delayed repair), UA (if +UTI → fistula present), sacral XR/spine USG or MRI (eval for associated spinal/sacral anomalies); rx: if < 1 cm distance → primary repair w/ cutback anoplasty; if > 1 cm distance → colostomy, refer for delayed repair w/ PSARP (posterior sagittal anorectoplasty); if +urinary fistula will need takedown

Testicular torsion – dx: USG w/ doppler; rx: manual detorsion (direction of rotation = opening a book, obtain repeat USG w/ doppler after), elective orchiopexy

Testicular mass – dx: labs (AFP/HCG/LDH), CXR, USG scrotum, CTAP; rx: transinguinal orchiectomy, then: 1) seminoma (normal AFP, usually normal HCG): if retroperitoneal LNs negative on CTAP → XRT, if retroperitoneal LNs positive on CTAP → XRT + add platinum-based chemo and mediastinal XRT 2) nonseminomas (elevated AFP and/or HCG): if LNs negative → RPLND w/ postop chemo, if LNs positive → neoadjuvant chemo followed by RPLND

Undescended testes – HCG stim test, if LH/FSH remain high and testosterone low → implies anorchia (no sx); if undescended testes, localize by exam/USG/MRI and perform orchiopexy if not down by 1-2 yrs age

OPERATIVE GUIDE

GENERAL TIPS

Before describing the operation go over the following: preoperative antibiotic or bowel prep prn, anesthesia strategy (ie. general vs local), mention invasive monitors prn, positioning

Remember preparatory intraop procedures (ex. EGD, rigid proctoscopy, bronch)

Examine for liver mets/peritoneal carcinomatosis in abdominal cancer cases and biopsy prn prior to resection

Don't forget to do frozen section if needed and re-resect for margin prn

Orient specimen for pathologist

Remember to heparinize before clamping vessels

Check your work (ex. leak tests, repeat EGD/bronch)

Place appropriate drains

Perform adjunctive procedures (ex. jejunostomy tube, cholangiogram) as indicated

HEAD/NECK

Parotidectomy – divide EJV, identify posterior belly of digastric @ mastoid, identify main trunk of facial nerve, dissect superficial lobe of parotid from nerve, divide Stensen's duct

Deep parotidectomy – dissect facial nerve off deep lobe, divide posterior facial vein, superficial temporal a/v, internal maxillary a/v, external carotid a/v

Central LND - boundaries: brachiocephalic artery (inferior) to hyoid bone (superior), between common carotid arteries (lateral) = pretracheal/prelaryngeal/paratracheal LNs = level VI LNs.

Sistrunk procedure – incision slightly higher than thyroidectomy, dissect out cyst/track, excise entirety including portion of hyoid bone up to base of tongue, drain

Thyroid lobectomy – divide platysma/strap muscles, divide middle thyroid vein, ligate superior vessels close to gland, identify and preserve RLN and parathyroid glands, ligate inferior vessels once RLN identified, dissect thyroid off trachea and divide at isthmus. Repeat lobectomy on other side if total thyroid indicated (unless RLN injury suspected → then abort).

Parathyroidectomy (focused exploration) - resect abnormal gland and measure intraop PTH levels (should drop by 50% from the higher of 2 values: baseline PTH or PTH at 0 minutes following resection) → if does not drop appropriately proceed with 4 gland exploration

Parathyroidectomy (4-gland exploration) - identify 4 glands, if find adenoma remove and consider sending intraop PTH levels. If no adenoma or suspect hyperplasia instead, biopsy to confirm → subtotal parathyroidectomy (remove 3.5 glands, remove the 0.5 gland first to make sure remaining 0.5 is viable) or total parathyroidectomy w/ reimplantation (brachioradialis or SCM)

RND/MRND –incision going from vertically along anterior border of SCM then curves posteriorly to lateral clavicle; develop skin flaps (laterally to border of trapezius; medially to strap muscles); borders of dissection: medial – strap muscles, lateral – trapezius, superior – mandible, inferior – clavicle; first divide attachment of SCM to sternum/clavicle inferiorly, then divide the following structures going laterally to medially (EJV, SAN, posterior belly of omohyoid, IJV), then reflect tissue upwards and dissect from inferior to superior to clear all lymph tissue from around IJV(avoid phenic n, vagus n, common carotid a), move anteriorly and remove the submandibular gland (need to divide salivary duct; avoid lingual and hypoglossal n), divide anterior belly of omohyoid and superior ends of IJV/SCM/SAN/EJV, remove specimen, place drain, close; MRND – preserves one or more of the following (SAN, IJV, SCM)

Tracheostomy – between 2nd and 3rd rings

Cricothyroidotomy – NOT in kids; convert to trach within 24 hrs

BREAST/SOFT TISSUE

FNA – 22ga needle, multiple passes on suction without withdrawing, then stop suction and withdraw, expel onto 2 slides, prep w/ 95% etoh

Core needle bx – 14 ga needle

Lumpectomy – remember to get needle localization before, remember to orient specimen

Sentinel lymph node bx – inject radionuclide tracer (technetium sulfur colloid) 3-24 hr before, do lymphoscintigraphy (esp if primary in trunk) to identify draining nodal basin(s), inject methylene blue into area of tumor, resect nodes that are EITHER hot or blue. Achieve < 10% of peak count w/ dissection (resect any LN w/ > 10% of count of hottest SLN). If cannot find SLN → proceed with complete regional LND. If performing in conjunction w/ lumpectomy or mastectomy, do SLN bx BEFORE breast resection.

MRM – total mastectomy + ALND; borders: clavicle, inframam crease, sternum, lat dorsi

ALND – borders: axillary vein, pec major, lat dorsi, chest wall, avoid long thoracic/thoracodorsal nerves; levels I-II (lateral to and underneath pec minor) in breast ca, levels I-III (level III = medial to pec minor) in melanoma

Superficial inguinal lymphadenectomy – incision: S-shaped - start medial/cephalad to anterior superior iliac spine, runs caudal to below inguinal crease, then run medial until reaching femoral vein, turn caudal for another 5 cm; clear femoral triangle - borders: inguinal ligament (superior), sartorius (lateral), adductor longus (medial), floor = femoral vessels; consider transposing sartorius to protect femoral vessels

Deep inguinal (pelvic) lymphadenectomy – divide inguinal ligament, divide external oblique, internal oblique, transversalis, expose iliac vessels while keeping peritoneum intact, clear space b/t internal and external iliac arteries, floor=obturator membrane overlying the foramen, close layers, remember to reconstruct inguinal ligament

Wide local excision – down to fascia, orient specimen

LUNG

Lobectomy – thoracotomy 5th ICS, identify phrenic nerve, divide inferior pulmonary ligament, divide branches of pulmonary artery to appropriate lobe, identify superior and inferior pulmonary veins + isolate/divide appropriate vein, isolate/divide appropriate bronchus (clamp and have anesthesia insufflate before dividing to confirm correct bronchus and not mainstem), divide fissure, leave chest tube

Pneumonectomy – thoracotomy 5th ICS, identify phrenic nerve, divide inferior pulmonary ligament, divide main PA, divide superior and inferior pulmonary veins, divide main stem bronchus, place intercostal muscle flap, leave chest tube w/ balanced drainage

Mediastinoscopy – cervical incision 1 finger breadth above sternal notch, divide platysma transversely, divide strap muscles in midline, expose pretracheal fascia and incise, bluntly dissect pretracheal space into mediastinum w/ finger, insert mediastinoscope, identify LNs at stations 2R, 2L,4R, 4L, 7 and bx (2 = proximal paratracheal, 4 = distal paratracheal, 7 = subcarinal – which count as ipsilateral LNs), avoid PA (above you), azygos (down and to the right), esophagus (under level7), RLN (down and to the left), send for frozen section, pack for hemostasis, then close

ESOPHAGUS/STOMACH

Ivor-Lewis esophagogastrectomy – enter abdomen, kocher maneuver, divide gastrocolic ligament (preserve gastroepiploic arteries), divide short gastrics, divide L gastric artery, start tubularizing stomach from below, pyloromyotomy, J tube, close and flip, R 5th ICS thoracotomy, dissect out esophagus, divide it proximally, place pursestring on proximal end w/ anvil for EEA, pull up stomach through hiatus, deploy EEA tip through gastrostomy (away from site of future conduit) and join w/ anvil, complete gastric conduit w/ stapler from above (exclude gastrotomy site), chest tube

Exposure of cervical esophagus – incision parallel and anterior to SCM, divide platysma, retract SCM laterally, divide middle thyroid vein and retract thyroid medially, encircle esophagus (avoid RLN) if necessary

Colon interposition – remember preop angio/bowel prep, dissect out esophagus via thoracotomy (either L or R) but leave in place, enter abdomen, take down both flexures, bulldogs to test blood supply, if basing off L colic artery then divide middle colic artery proximally and preserve marginal artery, divide colon proximally enough to obtain necessary length, divide colon distal to L colic, reconnect colon, divide GE junction/prox stomach, suture prox conduit to distal esophagus (to be able to pull up later), expose cervical esophagus, pass conduit up anatomically by pulling esophagus up via neck incision, resect esophagus, perform esophagocolonic (prox) and cologastric (dist) anastomoses, pyloromyotomy, J tube; if using substernal path of conduit will need clavicular head resection

Paraesophageal hernia repair (transabdominal) – reduce hernia, resect hernia sac, collis gastroplasty for short esophagus (remember to place bougie prior, need 1-2 cm length of esophagus in abdomen), close hiatal defect posteriorly (can use surgisys or other biologic mesh prn), perform fundoplication (Nissen = 360, Toupet = posterior 180, Dor = anterior 180) unless poor esophageal motility

Zenker's – expose cervical esophagus (see above), dissect out diverticulum, divide cricopharyngeus for a distance 5-6 cm caudal from where diverticulum is, staple diverticulum w 60Fr bougie in place, leave drain

Graham patch – create tongue of omentum, place interrupted 3-0 silk sutures w/ plan to reapproximate perforation, secure omentum into perf by tying these sutures on top of it, consider JP drain, lavage abdomen

Laparoscopic Nissen fundoplication – take down gastrohepatic ligament, dissect out hiatus (see both diaphragmatic crura, pass dissector behind esophagus), take short gastric arteries, mobilize fundus and "shoeshine" behind esophagus, remember bougie prior to closing any hiatal defect and creating the fundoplication

Heller myotomy – extend myotomy distally for no more than 1 cm past GE junction, extend myotomy proximally until reaching dilated esophagus, total length of myotomy = 5-7 cm, do post myotomy EGD, fill upper abdomen w saline to watch for bubbles/ensure mucosal integrity

Pyloroplasty – longitudinal incision @ pylorus, close transversely in 2 layers

Pyloric exclusion – gastrotomy, oversew pylorus w/ PDS or prolene (will open up later on its own), also do gastrojejunostomy

Vagotomy – mobilize L liver, clear all tissue around esophagus, resect section of vagus from both trunks and send for frozen, do drainage procedure (pyloroplasty, antrectomy, or G-J)

Proximal/parietal cell vagotomy – isolate both vagus nerves, identify anterior and posterior nerves of Latarjet (going to antrum), divide all branches going between vagus and stomach but spare latarjet/main trunk vagus, no drainage procedure needed, reapproximate peritoneum over lesser curvature

Subtotal gastrectomy (for ca) – divide gastrocolic ligament and perform omentectomy, elevate stomach and divide L gastric artery, move down towards R gastric artery, take LNs along common hepatic, divide R gastric, Kocher, divide duodenum, divide proximal stomach (50% resection = 2nd vein on lesser curve), need 8 cm margin prox, D1 dissection = perigastric, suprapyloric/infrapyloric, D2=celiac, hepatic, splenic

Antrectomy (for PUD) - do not need to divide R and L gastric arteries at origin, rather, divide gastric and gastroepiploic arcades where resection is to be done (50% gastrectomy),

Total gastrectomy – similar to subtotal but start distally and go proximally, divide entire blood supply, stapled anastomosis, w EEA transect 15 cm from treitz, but need 60 cm limb between esophagojejunostomy and jejunoojejunostomy to avoid bile reflux

Billroth I reconstruction – Kocher to mobilize duodenum, end-to-end gastroduodenostomy, avoid in cancer

Billroth II reconstruction – side-to-side gastrojejunostomy

SMALL BOWEL/LARGE BOWEL/ANUS
SBR – remember to close mesentery
Lap appendectomy – ports: umbilical, suprapubic, LLQ

Open appendectomy – RLQ incision, muscle splitting, enter peritoneum, perform appy, cauterize mucosa after dividing, purse-string and invert base of appendix

Transduodenal diverticulectomy – kocher, duodenotomy, identify ampulla of vater, identify diverticulum, evert into duodenum and transect, repair in 2 layers, close duodenotomy, place drain

R hemicolectomy – take down hepatic flexure, identify ureter, divide ileocecal/right colic and right branch of middle colic arteries (if hepatic flexure lesion/extended R hemicolectomy instead divide middle colic at its origin), resect/anastomose

Lap R hemicolectomy – 4 ports 5 mm (LUQ, RLQ, suprapubic, umbilical), divide ileocecal artery, dissect medial to lateral, visualize duodenum, place endoloop @ appendix, exteriorize via midline epigastric incision to resect/perform anastomosis

L hemicolectomy – usually needs xiphoid to pubis incision, take down splenic flexure, identify ureter, take IMA, resect/anastomose

Sigmoid colectomy – take down splenic flexure prn, identify ureter (consider preop ureteral stents if bulky lesion/diverticulitis); take IMA just distal to L colic, resect/anastomose

LAR – steps for L hemicolectomy, but prior to resecting bowel do total mesorectal excision (sharp dissection anterior to endopelvic fascia), need to incise Waldeyer's fascia posteriorly and Denonvillier's fascia anteriorly, anastomosis (can use EEA) +/- diverting ileostomy

Total colectomy – omentectomy, mobilize R colon, divide terminal ileum, mobilize L colon, divide mesentery, if subtotal divide at rectosigmoid junction and perform end ileostomy or ileorectal anastomosis, if total proctocolectomy do TME and perform either end ileostomy or mucosectomy with IPAA

APR – abdominal phase - do LAR , but close pelvic peritoneum, tack omentum into pelvis, bring out colostomy; perineal phase – close anus w/ pursestring, make elliptical incision around anus to perirectal fat, divide anococcygeal ligament, (posterior) , divide levators (lateral), divide tissue anterior (do not injure prostate or vagina), JP drain, close perineum

Total colectomy with proctomucosectomy and IPAA–mucosectomy 1st prone, then flip and do total colectomy, create J pouch (open ileum at midpoint of J and fire stapler once in each direction, then close with another staple load), bring down to anus and perform ileoanal anastomosis from below (single layer interrupted), then diverting loop ileostomy

Mucosectomy– prone jackknife; inject solution into submucosal plane immediately proximal to dentate line to separate mucosa from muscle, dissect mucosa from upper end of anal canal (distally) to rectum (proximally), purse string mucosa and resect, leaving muscle cuff; can also do this procedure from ABOVE

Loop ileostomy – conventional orientation: cephalad = proximal, caudad = distal SB; make transverse opening @ distal (non-functional end) + Brooke proximal end, place looped red rubber underneath

Transverse colostomy – R transverse abdominal incision @ epigastrium, divide greater omentum to expose colon

Ileostomy/colostomy reversal – incise skin around stoma, dissect out bowel from subcutaneous tissue/fascia, freshen edges + close stoma (or exclude ends w/ stapled anastomosis if enough mobility), close fascia, leave wound open

Hartmann's reversal – dissect out colon and rectum, take down splenic flexure, consider proctoscopy w/ insufflation if difficult to identify rectum, anastomosis

Cecostomy tube – RLQ incision, invert cecum around tube w/ 2 purse strings, then have tube exit skin above incision and secure

Hemorrhoidectomy – jackknife, inject local, hill-ferguson retractor, excise ellipses overlying R anterolateral/R posterolateral/L hemorrhoids no greater than 1.5 cm in diameter (otherwise can result in stenosis), close with locked chromic or vicryl

Perineal rectosigmoidectomy (Altemeier procedure) – jackknife, lonestar retractor, divide mucosa/muscle at the new "dentate line", take as much redundant rectosigmoid colon as possible by dividing mesentery, divide prox colon sharply, hand-sewn coloanal anastomosis

Lateral internal sphincterotomy (closed) – identify groove b/t internal and external sphincters, insert 11 blade into groove with tip to level of dentate line, rotate blade 90 degrees so cutting side towards mucosa, place finger on mucosa and cut through internal sphincter only (not mucosa), rupture remaining fibers w/ finger

Plication sphincteroplasty - anterior semicircular incision, expose internal sphincter, transverse perineal muscle (laterally), and levators (deep), then reapproximate levators and plicate (overlap) the internal sphincter and transverse perineal muscles

Presacral drain – curvilinear incision posterior to anus, enter presacral space, place penrose

HEPATOBILIARY/PANCREATIC

Choledochoduodenostomy – kocher maneuver, longitudinal incision in CBD, longitudinal incision in duodenum, "diamond" anastomosis, NO t-tube needed, don't forget chole, place drain

Roux-en-Y choledochojejunostomy – create roux limb 15 cm distal to ligament of treitz, bring up through mesocolon R of middle colic artery, end-to-side anastomosis with CBD, don't forget chole

Sphincteroplasty – kocher, perform choledochotomy and insert tube to identify ampulla, longitudinal duodenotomy over ampulla, place probe in ampulla and incise at 10-11 o'clock, place sutures to approximate duodenal and ductal mucosa, do this for 2 cm (to complete sphincterotomy) or the diameter of CBD (if residual stones/large CBD), if pancreatic duct stenosis → identify this orifice (5 o'clock) and perform ductoplasty, close duodenotomy, don't forget chole, place drain

Lap cholecystectomy – 4 ports: umbilicus, epigastric, RUQ x2; retract fundus laterally and cranially, obtain "critical view" (clear triangle of calot of fatty/fibrous tissue, separate GB from liver at infundibulum, see only 2 structures – cystic artery/duct – going to GB) prior to ligating

Cholecystectomy – R subcostal incision, pack away bowel/use bookwalter, top down dissection, ligate cystic duct/cystic artery, JP if possible bile leak

Cholangiogram – either via GB or cystic duct

R hepatectomy (segments 5-8) – divide falciform/triangular lig, divide gastrohepatic lig, chole, divide R hepatic duct/artery/portal vein, retract liver medially, divide small veins to IVC, divide R hepatic vein, divide parenchyma where demarcates (finger fracture or CUSA, clip arteries/veins/bile ducts, ABC for raw surface), ligate M hepatic vein, drain

Extended R hepatectomy (segments 4-8) – parenchymal division is at level of falciform ligament (take segment IV), use USG to make sure you avoid L portal vein

L hepatectomy (segments 1-4) – divide falciform/triangular lig, divide gastrohepatic lig, chole, divide L hepatic duct/artery/portal vein, divide parenchyma where demarcates, divide L hepatic vein, divide veins from IVC to caudate lobe (segment 1), drain

Lateral segmentectomy (segments 2-3) – avoid L hepatic vein by staying 1-2 cm left of falciform ligament

CBD exploration/choledochotomy/T tube placement – traction sutures either side, longitudinal incision, stone forceps / 4 Fr fogarty catheter, go distally and proximally into hepatic ducts, insert 10 Fr rubber catheter into duodenum to make sure you have cleared stones, don't forget chole; for T tube need rubber (NOT silicone) tube to be reactive, cut away opposite side of tube to facilitate removal, insert via choledochotomy and close around it with 4-0 PDS

Drainage of pancreatic cyst – bx wall, use permanent suture (cystgastrostomy if adjacent to stomach, cystjejunostomy if not)

Resection of Klatskin's tumor – chole, identify R and L hepatic ducts / CBD, confirm no invasion of PV, divide proximally / distally, send for frozen section to determine margin, complete anastomoses (R and L hepaticojej + jejunojej) over preexisting transhepatic drains brought out through dome of liver / skin, leave drains at each of exit sites @ dome of liver

Pancreatic tumor enucleation – IOUS to identify tumor, give IV secretin if concern for leak, tack omentum down to area after enucleation, drain

Puestow – open PD longitudinally, clear of calculi, side to side anastomosis to Roux limb of jejunum, place drain

Whipple – explore for mets, chole, kocher, confirm resectability (free from portal vein / SMV), dissect portal triad, ligate GDA and divide CBD after confirming no replaced RHA, divide antrum (classic Whipple) or duodenum (pylorus-sparing Whipple), place sutures at inferior / superior borders of pancreas distal and proximal to where you will transect, transect and ligate bleeders, free uncinate from SMA, free ligament of treitz and divide jejunum to remove specimen, bring roux-limb up and perform pancreaticojejunostomy in 2 layers, hepaticojejunostomy / gastrojejunostomy in 1 layer, place G tube and possible J tube, drain, remember FROZEN SECTION

Distal pancreatectomy – identify tumor (USG if necessary), mobilize spleen (divide short gastric arteries, splenorenal ligament), divide splenic artery / vein, divide pancreas with stapler, leave drain

Total pancreatectomy – kocher, confirm resectability (free from portal vein / SMV), divide antrum, divide GDA / CBD, then mobilize spleen / tail of pancreas, divide splenic artery / vein, free uncinate from SMA, free ligament of treitz and divide jejunum, bring roux-limb up and perform hepaticjej, gastrojej, place G tube and possible J tube, drain

SPLEEN/ADRENAL

Elective splenectomy – midline or L subcostal incision, divide short gastric arteries, ligate splenic artery, divide splenorenal/splenocolic ligament when mobilizing spleen, after mobilizing spleen place lap pad behind, divide splenic artery/vein, check for accessory spleens – most commonly in splenic hilum, other sites = splenocolic, splenorenal, gastrosplenic ligaments, tail of pancreas, SB mesentery

Trauma splenectomy –midline incision, mobilize spleen 1st, control bleeding w/ manual pressure @ vessels, ligate artery/vein, then take short gastric

Lap splenectomy – slight R lateral decubitus, 4 ports (from R to L: epigastrium, mid clavicular line below costal margin, anterior axillary line, mid axillary line), same steps as open

R adrenalectomy – mobilize R colon, Kocher, mobilize R liver, expose adrenal, ligate adrenal vein 1st, then ligate all other vessels going to it

L adrenalectomy – mobilize spleen/pancreas, stay anterior to gerota's fascia/kidney, expose adrenal, ligate adrenal vein 1st, then other vessels

Lap adrenalectomy–lateral decubitus position, 4 ports (epigastrium, mid clavicular line below costal margin, 1 port medial, anterior axillary line, mid axillary line), same steps as open

HERNIA

Ventral hernia repair (underlay) – dissect hernia sac, reduce, reapproximate posterior sheath, place prolene mesh beneath muscle, close anterior sheath, relaxing incisions prn, drains

Lap ventral hernia repair – reduce hernia, use parietex mesh (polyester, dual sided), 5 cm overlap each side, place prolene sutures into mesh (used for transfascial fixation), roll up mesh and deploy in port, pass sutures through abdominal wall, tack edges

Lichtenstein hernia repair – divide external oblique, identify and isolate (or cut) ilioinguinal nerve, isolate spermatic cord, dissect and reduce direct and indirect hernia sacs, position and secure mesh (leave space for spermatic cord to pass through mesh), close in layers

Bassini repair – suture "triple layer" (tranversalis fascia, transversus abdominus, internal oblique) to inguinal ligament

Mcvay repair – suture triple layer to Cooper's ligament, need transition stitch to inguinal ligament when you reach the femoral vein, remember relaxing incision @ rectus

Lap inguinal hernia repair (TEPP) – don't forget foley before, periumbilical incision, enter preperitoneal space beneath anterior sheath R or L of midline (towards side of hernia), place and inflate dissecting balloon, then structural balloon, then place 5 mm ports x2 (suprapubic and midway between pubis and umbo), dissect hernia away from abdominal wall, place mesh, tack to pubic bone and anterosuperior to anterior superior iliac spine, make sure peritoneum does not slide underneath mesh when desufflating

VASCULAR

Open AAA repair (transabdominal) – midline incision, retract transverse colon cephalad, eviscerate small bowel to R, enter RP to expose aorta, obtain proximal control @ aorta, distal control @ common iliacs, heparinize then clamp, open aneurysm and oversew lumbar arteries/IMA, perform proximal/distal anastomosis (tube graft if iliacs OK, bifurcated graft if aneurysmal), deair/flash both proximally/distally prior to tying down suture, release clamps, close aneurysm sac around graft

Open AAA repair (retroperitoneal) - torso in R lateral decubitus, hips rotated back as flat as possible, incision from L 11th rib to rectus, pack peritoneal sac away medially, expose aorta (usually mobilize L kidney also); if repairing TAAA go higher - type I-II $\rightarrow$ 6th ICS, III $\rightarrow$ 7th or 8th, IV $\rightarrow$ 9th

Ruptured AAA repair – prep and drape before induction of anesthesia, no heparin, get supraceliac control 1st, then control iliacs, reposition clamp at infrarenal position, then perform AAA repair

Cross clamping aorta (supraceliac/intraabdominal) – mobilize left lobe of liver and retract cranially and to R, retract esophagus to L (NGT may be useful), divide R diaphragmatic crus prn, place clamp or use T-bar to get control

Aortoenteric fistula – if pt stable – perform axillobifemoral bypass first, then enter abdomen to resect graft/oversew aorta; if pt unstable – resect graft first, return to OR 1 day later to perform axillobifemoral bypass

Aortobifemoralbypass – expose aorta, bilateral femoral vessels, heparinize, then clamp prox aorta/bilat common iliacs/IMA and complete beveled end-to-side anastomosis of bifurcated graft, tunnel each end of graft to femoral, clamp CFA/SFA/profunda and perform anastomosis

Axillofemoral bypass – anastomosis to proximal axillary artery (medial to pec minor) to reduce dehiscence risk; pass graft between pec major and minor to lateral chest wall; fem-fem graft as distal as possible on axillofemoral graft (use ring supported PTFE – 10 mm ax-fem and 8 mm fem-fem in large people; 8 mm and 6 mm in small)

CEA – divide facial vein, expose/loop ICA/CCA/ECA, don't forget heparin, clamp (InternalCommonExternal – ICE – in that order), place shunt, endarterectomy, tack ends of plaque prn, flush, close w/ dacron patch; to get better exposure if high carotid lesion: 1) nasotracheal intubation 2) divide posterior belly digastric 3) resect styloid 4) subluxation of mandible (OMFS consult) 5) osteotomy of mandible (OMFS consult)

Below knee fasciotomy – medial incision 1 cm posterior to tibia (avoid saphenous vein), open up deep and superficial compartments, lateral incision between tibia and fibula (avoid superficial peroneal nerve), open up anterior and lateral compartments, can vac wounds

Above knee fasciotomy – anterolateral skin incision along iliotibial tract, open fascia over vastus lateralis, open intermuscular septum; check pressure in medial compartment, if still elevated make incision in skin/fascia overlying adductors

Lower extremity artery exposures - posterior tibial - separate gastroc/soleus, runs between PT and flex digitorum longus muscles; anterior tibial - incision 2 cm lateral to tibia, divide fascia overlying anterior compartment, separate AT and extensor digitorum longus; dorsalis pedis - incision 2 cm lateral to extensor hallucis longus; prox $2/3^{rd}$ peroneal artery - medial; distal $1/3^{rd}$ peroneal artery – lateral over fibula w/ excision of segment of fibula; profunda femoris – vertical groin incision, ligate lateral femoral circumflex vein

Visceral rotation - **Cattel** (mobilize R colon/Kocher)→ exposes IVC, R renal hilum, R iliac artery; **Mattox** (L colon, spleen, +/- L kidney)→ exposes SMA, L renal hilum, IMA, L iliac (to remember names, C is before M, right is proximal to left)

Visceral artery exposures – celiac – via lesser sac or Cattel maneuver; SMA – elevate transverse mesocolon, incise peritoneum at base over pulse; IMA – trace IMA to aorta, incise peritoneum; R renal artery – Cattel maneuver; L renal artery - Mattox maneuver or divide treitz/mobilize duodenum, incise peritoneum beneath pancreas towards left, retract vein cranially

Vertebral artery exposure – supraclavicular incision, divide clavicular head of SCM, retract IJV medially, protect phrenic and divide anterior scalene, protect thoracic duct, divide thyrocervical trunk branches prn, divide vertebral vein

Upper extremity artery exposures - L subclavian via L anterolateral thoracotomy; R subclavian or innominate arteries via sternotomy w R cervical extension; prox brachial artery w/ longitudinal incision between biceps and triceps in bicipital groove; dist brachial artery and bifurcation w/ longitudinal incision in antecubital fossa distal to elbow crease, divide bicipital aponeurosis

Forearm fasciotomy – volar incision - "lazy S", need to release carpal tunnel lig; dorsal incision – straight, need to release dorsal and mobile wad compartments

Portocaval shunt – kocher to expose IVC, isolate and expose contents of hepatoduodenal ligament, ellipse out segments of vein to be anastomosed (should be as long as portal vein is wide); can also perform end-to-side portocaval, H type portocaval (w/ graft), or mesocaval shunts (use SMV)

Distal splenorenal (Warren) shunt – omentectomy, expose inferior border of pancreas and identify splenic vein, ligate IMV, expose L renal vein and ligate adrenal and gonadal, then disconnect splenic vein from SMV and perform end-to-side anastomosis (distal end of splenic vein to renal vein); classic shunt is proximal end of splenic vein to renal + splenectomy

PEDS/UROLOGY/GYN/MISCELLANEOUS

Meckel's diverticulectomy – incidental/asymptomatic →diverticulectomy; symptomatic → SBR

EA/TEF repair – R thoracotomy, divide azygos, divide fistula, primary reanastomosis, flap to tracheal suture line if present, NGT, chest tube

Pyloromyotomy– transverse upper abdominal incision, deliver greater curve of stomach, 1-2 cm incision through serosa/muscle, confirm no perforation; postop – progressive increase in feeding starting 6 hrs after operation (15 cc, then 30 cc)

Ladd's procedure – detorsion of volvulus, broaden mesentery, division of Ladd's bands crossing duodenum, appendectomy, pexy duodenum/SB on R and large bowel on L

Radical orchiectomy – inguinal incision, approach spermatic cord as you would in hernia repair, protect ilioinguinal nerve, deliver testicle, divide gubernaculum (=scrotal ligament, tethers testicle in place), divide spermatic cord (vas and vascular supply separately), place testicular prosthesis

Hydrocele repair – make incision vertically on anterior surface of scrotum, isolate hydrocele with testicle/spermatic cord completely from scrotum, open hydrocele sac and excise redundant part, close posteriorly (everting it)

Salpingectomy – take mesosalpinx close to tube to avoid devascularizing ovary

Salpingoooopherectomy – take entire mesentery of ovary/tube

TAH – identify ureter, take ovarian vessels (if doing BSO), take uterine vessels, divide uterus, close vagina/cervix

Placement of Minnesota tube – pass tube into stomach, inflate balloon by 15 ml, AXR to confirm, then blow up to 500 ml, pull back and attach to weight/helmet to tamponade, aspirate esophageal port, then inflate it to 30 mm Hg, leave x24h, then deflate and EGD

DPL – positive if >100000 rbc (blunt), > 10000 rbc (penetrating), >500 wbc, gross blood, bile, food, use 15 cc/kg NS in child vs 1000 cc in adult, need return of 700 ml. Above umbilicus if pregnant or pelvic fx, otherwise infraumbilical.

FAST – 4 views: pericardium, hepatorenal fossa, splenic fossa, pelvis

Pericardiocentesis – 18 gauge spinal needle, start on L side of xiphoid pointing needle toward shoulder, 45 deg angle to skin, aspirate until you get fluid, if get air then aim more medially and assume PTX, if bloody then inspect → if clots, then blood was likely 2/2 injury sustained during procedure; if does not clot, then true hemopericardium from prior injury (if blood is exposed to pericardial fluid then it will not clot)

Subxiphoid window – midline subxiphoid incision, resect xiphoid, grasp pericardium w/ allis and incise, resect quarter-sized piece

ED thoracotomy – L thoracotomy from sternum to bed, extend across sternum and to R prn (ligate mammary vessels), pericardiotomy + repair heart prn, open cardiac massage + defibrillate prn, x-clamp aorta, evacuate bronchovenous air/clamp hilum if needed (aspirate from LV/LA/arch)

Trauma laparotomy – prep from neck to knees, incision from xiphoid to pubis, pack 4 quadrants, then run SB/LB bowel and clamp enterotomies, then go back to unpack each quadrant/address bleeding injuries, then repair bowel injuries

ABBREVIATION GUIDE

Ab – antibodies

ABC – airway, breathing, circulation or argon beam coagulator

Abx - antibiotics

AC - adriamycin/cyclophosphamide

ALND - axillary lymph node dissection

AT - anterior tibial artery or muscle

BAO - basal acid output

BCC - basal cell carcinoma

BCT - breast conserving therapy

BE - Barrett's esophagus

Bx – bx

Ca – cancer

C/b – complicated by

CBD - common bile duct

CBE - clinical breast exam

CD - Crohn's disease

CEA – carotid endarterectomy

CFA - common femoral artery

CHD - common hepatic duct

CHOP - cyclophosphamide, adriamycin, vincristine, prednisone

CLND - central lymph node dissection

Comps - complications

CPP – cerebral perfusion pressure

CRC – colorectal cancer

CRI - chronic renal insufficiency

CTNCAP - CT scan of neck/chest/abdomen/pelvis

Cx - culture

DCIS - ductal carcinoma in situ

DRE - digital rectal exam

DTA - descending thoracic aneurysm

Dx – diagnosis

Dz - disease

EJV - external jugular vein

Esp - especially

ETT – endotracheal tube

EUS - endoscopic ultrasound

FAC - 5-FU/adriamycin/cyclophosphamide

FTSG – full thickness skin graft

Fx – fracture

GEJ - gastroesophageal junction

GOO - gastric outlet obstruction

HD – hemodialysis or hemodynamic(ally)

HFOV - high frequency oscillatory ventilation

HGD - high grade dysplasia

HOP - head of pancreas

HPT – hyperparathyroidism

Hx – history

IABP – intraaortic balloon pump

ICS - intercostal space

IFN – interferon

IJV - internal jugular vein

IOUS - intraoperative ultrasound

LAN - lymphadenopathy

LCIS - lobular carcinoma in situ

LGD - low grade dysplasia

LN – lymph node

MAP – mean arterial pressure

Med - medication or mediastinoscopy

MRM – modified radical mastectomy

MRND - modified radical neck dissection

NAC - nipple-areolar complex

NTG – nitroglycerin

OCP - oral contraceptives

OLT - orthotopic liver transplant

PAO - peak acid output

PD - pancreatic duct

PE – physical exam or pulmonary embolism

PNA – pneumonia

Prox – proximal

PT - posterior tibial artery or muscle

PTC - papillary thyroid cancer or percutaneous transhepatic cholangiogram (catheter)

PTX – pneumothorax

PUD - peptic ulcer disease

PV - portal vein

PVD - peripheral vascular disease

RAIU - radioactive iodine uptake

RLN - recurrent laryngeal nerve

RND - radical neck dissection

RP – retroperitoneal

RPLND – retroperitoneal lymph node dissection

RUG - retrograde urehtrogram

Rx - treatment

RYGJ - Roux-en-Y gastrojejunostomy

RYHJ - Roux-en-Y hepaticojejunostomy

RYPJ – Roux-en-Y pancreaticojejunostomy

SAN - spinal accessory nerve

SAO - stimulated acid output

SB - small bowel

SBR - small bowel resection

SCC - squamous cell carcinoma

SCM - sternocleidomastoid

SEPS - subfascial endoscopic perforator surgery

SFA - superficial femoral artery

SLNBx - sentinel lymph node bx

STSG – split thickness skin graft

SVS - selective venous sampling

Sx – surgery

T+C – type and cross

TAAA - thoracoabdominal aortic aneurysm

TAC - taxotere/adriamycin/cyclophosphamide

TACE - transarterial catheter embolization

TBSA – total body surface area

TC - taxotere/cyclophosphamide

Tg - thyroglobulin

TM - total mastectomy

UC - ulcerative coliits

UOP - urine output

UPJ – ureteropelvic junction

USG – ultrasound

V + A - vagotomy + antrectomy

V + P - vagotomy + pyloroplasty

WLE - wide local excision

WPW - Wollf-Parkinson-White syndrome

XRT – radiation therapy

Z-E - Zollinger-Ellison syndrome

2906422R10036

Made in the USA
San Bernardino, CA
16 June 2013